EATING DISORDERS

ALSO BY TANIA HELLER, M.D.,
AND FROM MCFARLAND

*Pregnant! What Can I Do?
A Guide for Teenagers* (2002)

EATING DISORDERS

A Handbook for Teens, Families and Teachers

Tania Heller, M.D.

McFarland & Company, Inc., Publishers
Jefferson, North Carolina, and London

LIBRARY OF CONGRESS CATALOGUING-IN-PUBLICATION DATA

Heller, Tania, 1958–
    Eating disorders : a handbook for teens, families and teachers /
Tania Heller
      p.   cm.
    Includes bibliographical references and index.

    ISBN 0-7864-1478-2 (softcover : 50# alkaline paper)

    1. Anorexia nervosa—Handbooks, manuals, etc. 2. Eating
disorders in adolescence—Handbooks, manuals, etc. I. Title.
RC552.A5H45 2003
616.85'26—dc21   2003005736

British Library cataloguing data are available

Cover art ©2003 Artville

Manufactured in the United States of America

McFarland & Company, Inc., Publishers
  Box 611, Jefferson, North Carolina 28640
    www.mcfarlandpub.com

To all the young men and women struggling with eating disorders
and to their families who suffer with them.
Although the road to recovery can seem endless at times,
I hope you never lose faith.

Acknowledgments

I am very grateful to a large number of people who have helped make this book a possibility. Thanks to my family—Sam, Daniel, Ariel, Izzy, Zelda, Fay, Leon, Loren, Gabi and Ben—for their love and understanding. Thank you to psychiatrist and author Dr. E. James Lieberman for his encouragement; and to Karen Weinstein for her good advice over the years.

I'd also like to mention my appreciation for the young men and women who so generously shared their life stories, struggles and triumphs with me. (Names and identifying characteristics have been changed to maintain confidentiality.) I have faith that their courage will give hope and strength to others suffering from these difficult illnesses.

Contents

Preface

I have watched too many patients and families struggle with anorexia nervosa, bulimia nervosa, binge-eating disorder and numerous undefined eating disorders—illnesses that should be preventable. After seeing both the physical and psychological scars, I felt compelled to both write and do something about eating disorders.

In this book I will talk about these illnesses. I will also discuss body dysmorphia, and eating disorders in men as well as in women. I will talk about the warning signs of eating disorders, why people develop these disorders, and the function the disorders serve. Throughout, I will emphasize prevention, because prevention is far easier than treatment.

Although a relatively small percentage of teenage girls and boys develop classic anorexia nervosa or bulimia nervosa, many more young people have atypical eating disorders with symptoms such as severely restricting calories and being preoccupied with food and body weight. These people, too, are at risk for serious medical and psychological problems and also deserve our attention.

In the book I have also included a chapter on adolescent obesity. As a pediatrician, I have been seeing a new group of patients over the last few years. Many children and teenagers have come in with obesity-related illnesses, such as Type 2 diabetes, the type we usually see only in adults who are overweight. This is a preventable disease, usually related to diet and lifestyle habits. In our society, food is more processed, often laden with sugars and fats, and is often eaten on the run or at drive-through restaurants. Children, teenagers and adults are more sedentary, spending their time in front of computers, television sets, and video games, instead of exercising outdoors. The price they often pay is obesity, with all its complications. Although adolescent obesity is not formally classified as an eating disorder, I have included a chapter on the subject because a number of people with obesity have binge-eating disorder, which is an eating disorder, and because obesity is a common, serious and treatable nutritional problem among teenagers.

I wrote this book primarily for young people who are either eager to learn more about eating disorders and obesity, or who are themselves struggling with these problems. To them I say: Your teenage years are years of enormous growth, development and change in all sorts of ways. This transition time can be difficult, but at the same time it can be wonderful. It's a time when you need to start taking responsibility for yourself, and that includes your health. It's never too late to begin a healthier lifestyle. I hope this book encourages you to do so.

1

No Age Barriers

Long before I knew that I would be involved in the field of eating disorders, I encountered people and patients who affected me deeply, and who I will always remember. Perhaps they were the ones who inspired me to learn more about these illnesses, seek out new ways to help patients and their families, and spread the word about how we as a society can prevent eating disorders.

There are no age barriers to these illnesses. They can affect everyone from very young children to mature adults, as the following stories will show.

Personal Stories

Anna's Story

Anna sat on the examining table while her mother recounted her meals from the previous day. It didn't take long at all: a plain piece of toast for breakfast, an apple for lunch, and half a fat-free yogurt and a banana for dinner. It was clear that Anna did not want to be there. "I almost finished the yogurt!" she told her mother indignantly, and then turned to me: "I need to lose five more pounds for ballet." It was sad to see this young girl already beginning to waste away. Anna was nine years old.

She had joined a dance group six months earlier. Her mother had been an excellent dancer, and she had hoped that Anna would follow in her footsteps. Unfortunately, Anna, the youngest in the group, already felt the pressures to stay thin, and was putting herself at great risk, both physically and emotionally. Her mother, who had witnessed her own sister's long struggle with anorexia nervosa, was ready to do whatever it took to help her daughter. The decision was made to temporarily put ballet lessons on hold and to begin family therapy.

Now, a few years later, although she has mild body image concerns, Anna has turned the corner and is able to enjoy the life of a happy healthy teenager.

RUTH'S STORY

No matter what time of day I went to the health club, Ruth was there. She was about 60 years old and exercised as vigorously as a 20-year-old. In the changing room I noticed her weighing herself before and after workouts. She became noticeably thinner every week, and I wondered how she had the stamina to keep running. In spite of this, there she was, week after week, weighing herself twice a session, until one day she was no longer there. I never saw Ruth again.

I have no information about what happened to Ruth, but some patients with severe chronic anorexia do die from their diseases, and I think that Ruth may have been one of them.

ALLISON'S STORY

Allison, a 32-year-old administrative assistant, struggles with body image concerns. She started restricting calories at the age of twelve. Allison doesn't remember a specific event that triggered her first diet, but she thinks there were a number of factors that caused her to be dissatisfied with her body. Her best friend was very thin and obsessed with her weight and shape. Allison wanted to be just like her. Also, her mother, who was thin, well-groomed, and appeared to be "perfect" in every way, believed that appearances were very important, and condoned dieting. To this day Allison is still hurt when the first thing her mom says to her is "You've gained a few pounds," or "You look good," or even "You look so thin." "I wish she would say 'Hi, how are you?' first," Allison said. Another problem was that Allison's grandmother would refer to her as "chubby," and then in the next breath offer her a piece of cake. Allison is still puzzled by this double standard. "When I look back at old photos, I wasn't even fat! I looked fine."

The dieting started gradually, but then as Allison began receiving compliments on her weight loss, she restricted more and more, until her calorie intake was dangerously low. She obsessed about food and her weight, and this took up so much of her time that she began withdrawing from social activities. By the age of 14, the young girl who used to be popular and social became unhappy and lonely. She began binge eating at the age of 15. Allison remembers going from one fast-food restaurant to another, and then hiding in her car and eating. She felt as if she had no one to turn to, so she used foods to comfort her. She spent large amounts of money on food. In spite of eating to the point of feeling sick, Allison could not make herself throw up, so she resorted to laxatives to try to get rid of the extra calories. Allison felt disgusted with herself after bingeing, and between binges she would punish herself by restricting her intake. She remembers eating fruit and yogurt and virtually nothing else for three months. Her weight fluctuated dramatically. The cycle continued with episodes of bingeing and laxative use, and then periods of dangerous dieting, until Allison was brought to the hospital in serious condition.

Today, after treatment, Allison is certainly happier than she was. Even though she is thin, she is still not completely comfortable with her body and with herself, but she does socialize more and enjoys her job and being with her friends. She finds that when she sticks to a routine of exercising for 30 minutes a day, she feels less worried about her weight.

Allison's prediction: "Until our society changes, and becomes accepting of women as they really are, nothing will change. Women will continue to develop eating disorders. There is too much pressure, and too much value placed on appearance."

Rita's Story

Rita's family moved to the United States from Africa when she was five years old. Her family didn't have a lot of money, so she had to live without many of the luxuries that her friends had grown accustomed to. Unlike her friends, she didn't spend much time going shopping or going to movies. She had a difficult childhood, which was made worse by the fact that her parents separated when she was nine. Her mother won custody, and Rita lived at home with her and with her grandparents.

There were struggles at home. Her mother was stressed from the responsibilities of being a single mom. Rita made a point of being out of the home as much as possible. As she began spending more time with her friends, she became exposed to a new culture, new ideas and a new value system. Although her family referred to her as "big-built," she was athletic, and so when she was fourteen she decided to join a modern dancing group. As she watched the girls around her, Rita noticed that they were all thinner than she was, and so she made up her mind to go on a diet. She restricted her calories for several days and was amazed to see that she had lost two pounds. She decided to continue dieting, but by the second week she became ravenous, and bought chocolates and cookies on the way home from school. This began Rita's dangerous cycle of bingeing and restricting, which eventually led this once social, active girl to become withdrawn and isolated.

It was once thought that eating disorders occurred almost exclusively in smart, accomplished, wealthy teenage girls. It has now become clear that eating disorders have no age, sex, or cultural boundaries. They affect adults, teenagers, and even young children. They affect the poor and the wealthy, and are now being diagnosed with increasing frequency in other cultures.

It is important that young people learn about eating disorders and their dangers at an early age. I believe that by becoming more aware of eating disorders, having knowledge about their warning signs, risk factors and complications, and knowing when and where to go for help, one can better protect oneself from the physical and emotional consequences of these illnesses.

2

What Are Eating Disorders?

Eating disorders are serious, potentially life-threatening illnesses that involve disturbances in eating habits and excessive concerns about body weight and shape. They are not simple behavior problems but are instead caused by a combination of biological, psychological and cultural factors.

A large percentage of teenage girls and boys are dissatisfied with their bodies and have a desire to be thinner, or in the case of boys, more muscular. In our Western culture, dieting and the pursuit of thinness has almost become the "norm." We are inundated with television images and magazine covers of very thin models, and are led to believe that being thin is synonymous with being healthy and successful.

Many factors, including genetics, personality, family, and culture, can set one up for a poor body image and obsessive dieting. Not everyone who diets or wishes to be thinner has an eating disorder. However, when thoughts about food and body shape consume someone's life, and when people base their entire self-image on how they look and what they eat, an eating disorder exists. Not only does health suffer from these disorders, but eventually so do activities, work and relationships.

A few statistics will show you how common these illnesses are:

- About 8 million Americans suffer from eating disorders.
- Approximately 1 million American males have an eating disorder.
- For women, the lifetime prevalence of anorexia nervosa is between 0.5 percent and 3.7 percent; for bulimia it is between 1.1 percent and 4.2 percent (according to the National Institute of Mental Health).
- About 2 percent of the population suffers from binge-eating disorder (BED), but BED affects up to 30 percent of obese patients seeking treatment for obesity.
- In addition to those people with classic eating disorders, many more suffer from atypical eating disorders.

The most commonly described eating disorders are anorexia nervosa. bulimia nervosa, and binge-eating disorder.

We are reading more and have learned more about anorexia nervosa these days, but it is not a new disease. Fasting among women has occurred for centuries. The earliest written reference to anorexia nervosa was in 1689, when Thomas Morton, an English physician, wrote about a case of "wasting disease of nervous origin." Anorexia nervosa was first described in the modern medical literature only in the 1870s, and even then not much was known about the disorder till a hundred years later.

An increase in the number of cases seems to have begun in the 1960s, and in 1983 the well-known singer Karen Carpenter died of the complications of an eating disorder. This brought eating disorders into the media spotlight. Bulimia nervosa was recognized as a distinct medical entity and named as such only in 1979.

Anorexia and bulimia have similarities in that they both begin with dieting and an attempt to lose weight. In anorexia this leads to continued dieting, longstanding weight loss and a semi-starvation state. In bulimia, the initial restrictive diet leads to breakthrough binge eating, a natural consequence of hunger and starvation. The individual may then resort to behaviors such as self-induced vomiting, laxative use or fasting in order to prevent weight gain.

In the case of anorexia, several factors keep the disorder going. These are known as *perpetuating factors*. The biological effects of starvation can be a powerful stimulant. Also, initially the person often gets positive reinforcement in the form of frequent compliments on the weight loss. Finally, anorexia becomes a way of life, a new identity and a means of coping. In the case of bulimia, the binge-purging cycle, which is initially triggered by hunger, is eventually triggered by other needs and mood, as well as by habit and probable autonomic (nervous system) conditioning.

People who have eating disorders can persuade themselves that they are doing something good. Here are some of the explanations I have heard:

• The eating disorder gives the person a sense of purpose and is something to focus on and to worry about.
• The disorder sometimes serves as a distraction from other problems.
• Losing weight may give a temporary feeling of accomplishment.
• The person often gets positive reinforcement about weight loss at first.
• Bingeing can be a way of coping with stress temporarily.

Of course, the negative effects far outweigh any perceived benefits. An eating disorder can

• lead to physical and psychological complications.
• cause loss of friends because of the person's isolation and preoccupation with food and weight.
• be associated with psychiatric conditions such as obsessions, depression and anxiety.
• exacerbate low self-esteem.
• produce negative effects on work, relationships and social life.
• last a long time, even a lifetime; eating disorders are chronic disorders.

Anorexia Nervosa

Anorexia nervosa is a serious, potentially life-threatening illness. Although only a small percentage of teenage girls develop classic anorexia nervosa, many more develop a milder form of the illness. Five to 10 percent of all individuals with anorexia are male.

Anorexia nervosa is an illness in which patients starve themselves in order to become thinner. Patients with anorexia nervosa severely restrict their intake of calories, resulting in the inability to maintain a healthy weight or grow normally. They are obsessed with becoming not only thin, but thinner and thinner, so that they are never satisfied with the degree of weight loss that they achieve. They have an intense fear of gaining weight, and a disturbance in body image, and they view themselves as fat in spite of being very thin or even emaciated. Instead of improving with weight loss, their body image usually gets worse.

Anorexia nervosa often begins with a diet, but people with anorexia differ from others who diet in that they never "come off their diet" and never achieve their goal, as their goal weight is constantly pushed lower and lower. It therefore appears that weight and being thin is not the only issue, as getting thin and losing weight does not relieve their stress or their obsession. Their intense fear of fat and gaining weight gradually escalates, along with their obsession about food and meal planning, and they start isolating themselves from friends and family. Once this disorder has set in, the perpetuating factors keep it going, and the behavior develops addictive qualities of its own.

Anorexia nervosa may give a person a sense of control over the world. The eating disorder is often used as a way to cope with negative emotions. The anorexic feels that if she can at least control her eating and her size, then she is exhibiting some mastery. In truth, she is not in control at all.

Anorexia is also about needs and feelings. People with anorexia deny their needs and suppress their feelings, even their need for food and their feelings of hunger. They may feel that they do not deserve pleasure. Something that happens when people starve is that they lose their capacity to enjoy life.

People who develop anorexia nervosa do not plan to become anorexic when they begin dieting. As they lose more weight, they may continue to see themselves as overweight, and set lower and lower weight goals. The process takes on a life of its own. It's ironic that people with anorexia feel that their ability to restrict food and lose weight gives them a sense of control over their lives, yet they have really lost control, and it is the eating disorder that has taken over their lives. An eating disorder is not all about food. It affects all aspects of a person's life, and affects not only sufferers but the people around them too.

Doctors use official criteria to decide whether a person has anorexia nervosa. These criteria are published in a book called *Diagnostic and Statistical Manual of Mental Disorders*. According to this book, the criteria for diagnosing anorexia nervosa are the following:

A. Refusal to maintain body weight at or above a minimally normal weight for age and height (e.g., weight loss leading to maintenance of body weight less than 85 percent of that expected; or failure to make expected weight gain during periods of growth, leading to body weight less than 85 percent of that expected).

B. Intense fear of gaining weight or becoming fat, even though underweight.

C. Disturbance in the way in which one's body weight or shape is experienced, undue influence of body weight or shape on self-evaluation, or denial of the seriousness of the current low body weight.

D. In postmenarcheal females, amenorrhea, i.e., the absence of at least three consecutive menstrual cycles. (A woman is considered to have amenorrhea if her periods occur only following hormone, e.g., estrogen, administration.)*

There are two recognized types of anorexia nervosa:

Restricting Type: during the current episode of Anorexia Nervosa, the person has not regularly engaged in binge-eating or purging behavior (i.e., self-induced vomiting or the misuse of laxatives, diuretics, or enemas)

Binge-Eating/Purging Type: during the current episode of Anorexia Nervosa, the person has regularly engaged in binge-eating or purging behavior (i.e., self-induced vomiting or the misuse of laxatives, diuretics, or enemas)*

In other words, a person with "restricting type" anorexia loses weight by eating very little and may or may not exercise excessively, while a person with "binge eating/purging type" not only restricts calories, but also binges and may vomit, or may use laxatives or pills, to control weight.

Because of starvation, the body "slows down" to conserve energy. This can result in serious health risks.

Symptoms of anorexia nervosa include:

• Weight loss (body fat may be significantly lower than normal)
• Denial of hunger (even though people with anorexia nervosa do experience it)
• Frequent weighing.

*Reprinted with permission from the Diagnostic and Statistical Manual of Mental Disorders, Fourth Edition, Text Revision. Copyright 2000 American Psychiatric Association.

   • Slow pulse and low blood pressure (due to slowing down of the body's functions)
   • Feeling cold or having cold hands and feet. (The body's metabolism slows down as it tries to conserve energy, and this can result in the individual feeling cold all the time.)

   • Fatigue, weakness
   • Constipation
   • Dry skin, dry hair
   • Dizziness or fainting
   • Loss of menstrual periods
   • Osteoporosis ("thinning" of the bones)
   • Difficulty concentrating or making decisions
   • Irritability or depression
   • Sleep disturbances
   • Sensitivity to criticism
   • Withdrawal from family and friends; isolation
   • Rigidity (The person may have great difficulty with any change in routine, and is usually very rigid about diet and meals, often eating almost the same menu every day.)
   • Obsession about food, including the preparation of food for others. (Some people with anorexia spend time and energy preparing elaborate meals for others, without eating any of the food themselves.)
   • Excessive exercising or excessive fidgeting
   • Difficulty sleeping

   Low self-esteem is present in people with anorexia nervosa, just as it is in the case of other eating disorders.
   Here are some stories of people with anorexia nervosa.

STACY'S STORY

   Until the age of fourteen Stacy would have been described as the perfect child. She was quiet, always listened to her parents, and was a straight A student. She had a fair number of friends with whom she rarely argued. She was tall, very pretty and neither too fat nor too thin. All in all it appeared as if Stacy had everything. However, nine months after her fourteenth birthday she was brought to me by her mother, who was concerned that in spite of an increase in her activity level, Stacy's appetite had decreased and she had been losing weight steadily. In addition, her periods, which had begun at age thirteen, had become irregular.

As I questioned Stacy further about what was going on, she reluctantly told me about her very controlling boyfriend, who regularly remarked that she was "chubby," even while she was losing weight rapidly, and who used threats to get her to "obey" him. After the first comment about her weight, Stacy had begun a diet, and now she felt compelled to continue the diet, in order to lose even more weight.

Stacy was referred to an eating disorder center right away, but had a difficult course at first. Her follow up was poor. She began vomiting in order to lose more weight, and had to be hospitalized when she lost seven more pounds in six days and became dehydrated. "If I gain any weight, I'll lose all control," Stacy told me, as she clung to her resolve.

After she was rehydrated and her nutrition was restored in hospital, she was started back on an outpatient program to further increase her weight and work on self-esteem issues. As Stacy became healthier her fear of gaining weight actually diminished. The last time I spoke to her, several years after her hospitalization, she was still doing well. Although she had a difficult course, which involved two hospitalizations and gall bladder surgery due to the development of gallstones, her outcome was better than some.

Not everyone with anorexia nervosa is as lucky. The mortality rate in anorexia is significant, both from the illness itself, and from suicide in the patients who become severely depressed.

BRENDA'S STORY

Brenda became unhappy with her weight and started dieting at the age of fourteen. Her best friend had moved out of the area the previous year and Brenda had recently moved to a new school in which she had trouble making friends. Both of these factors played a role in her feeling unhappy about herself, but the final straw was comparing herself to her classmates in gym class and believing that every one of them looked fitter and thinner than she did. Brenda was a healthy fourteen-year-old who was neither too fat nor too thin, but she began a diet, which was not unusual for girls of her age. What was unusual though, was that after she had lost five pounds, and had received several compliments, Brenda decided to continue dieting, eliminating more and more "bad" foods. She began by eliminating bread and butter, then eggs and meat, and then most fats and starches. Eventually her diet consisted of small amounts of fruits and vegetables and diet sodas. Her weight dropped rapidly at first, and when it began to plateau, she increased exercising, often running and biking daily.

Brenda was hospitalized once and also developed severe depression requiring medication. She is now followed by a physician, a therapist and a nutritionist and is recovering. She still struggles with body image issues, but feels happier. Brenda told me that participating in group sessions and being more involved socially and in her community helps most.

SHELLEY'S STORY

Shelley was a clever, popular child. She was not unhappy with her body, but did remember being self-conscious at times, particularly during co-ed swim class at school. After high school, Shelley left town to attend college, during which time she lived on campus in dorms. During her first month in college, a male friend she had not seen for a year remarked that she had gained a little weight. This innocent remark made a huge impact, and she began cutting down on her calories. Her restriction of food became more drastic over the next few months, as her weight dropped lower and lower. Eventually, Shelley's average daily intake consisted of nothing more than a bagel, fruit, cereal and diet soda.

Anorexia nervosa is not a passing phase or a condition you can snap out of. If you are suffering from anorexia, you may have had a relative or a friend tell you to "just eat" or to "get over it." These people usually mean well and may want to help, but their comments are neither helpful nor welcome.

Truthfully, although you may feel in control, most people with anorexia nervosa need help in order to recover. Without professional help, the prognosis is not good, and serious complications and even death can result from the illness. On the other hand, with early appropriate treatment, the outcome is very good.

Bulimia Nervosa

Bulimia is a serious eating disorder in which the person may be caught up in a dangerous cycle of binge eating and purging. Approximately 1 to 2 percent of teenage girls and young adult women develop classic bulimia nervosa, but the incidence can be much higher among college women. We used to think that bulimia occurred mostly in older adolescents, but we now see it in younger people too. About 10 percent of people with bulimia are male.

The word bulimia is derived from the Greek word meaning "ox hunger." The disorder was formally described in the medical literature only in the late 1970s, but this disorder, which is more common than anorexia, has probably existed for a long time.

The hallmark of bulimia is binge eating. People with bulimia usually eat an enormous amount of food in a short period of time. They can consume thousands or even tens of thousands of calories in one sitting. They do this in an automatic, out-of-control manner, and binges are followed by guilt and self-loathing. In order to get rid of the excess calories that they have taken in, they follow the binge with purging (self-induced vomiting, laxative or diuretic use), excessive exercise, or fasting. People suffering with bulimia are excessively concerned about body shape and weight, and have a great fear of gaining weight and becoming fat. Efforts to lose weight are usually unsuccessful, and patients with bulimia are usually of normal weight or slightly overweight. Some patients with bulimia have a history of anorexia nervosa.

Like anorexia, bulimia is not all about food, although it seems so to those suffering with the illness. Their thoughts are consumed by food, weight and planning binges. They eat to fulfill their need not only for food, but also their emotional needs and their loneliness. The cycle of bingeing and purging provides only temporary relief and does not lead to a sense of peace or accomplishment. In fact, people generally feel ashamed, and soon enough, to relieve their tension, they binge again. This leads to feelings of guilt and disgust and often a restriction of food intake, which sets them up for another binge. This is the so-called "binge-purge cycle." The person with bulimia has an underlying need or "hunger," but misidentifies it as a need for food.

Both anorexia and bulimia are associated with a low self-esteem, which worsens as these illnesses progress.

People with bulimia nervosa rely on others for approval. They are preoccupied with their body weight and shape. They begin dieting, which leads to feelings of hunger, which precipitates binge eating. To compensate for the binge, they diet or purge, to get rid of food and calories, only to repeat the cycle and binge again. Bingeing and purging is used as a substitute for dealing with emotions and as a way of coping with stress or dealing with disappointment. This cycle temporarily helps to regulate their mood, but in the long run sets them up for intense feelings of guilt, shame, and often depression. They have to plan the binges and often spend lots of money on food. They may find themselves telling lies to cover up their secret life, and relationships begin to suffer.

Purging is habit-forming. Remember that every patient caught in a binge-purge cycle began with just one purge. It starts out as a once-in-a-while event, perhaps to be able to eat a lot and still fit into a small size, but it quickly becomes a habit which is difficult to break.

Like anorexia nervosa, bulimia nervosa is diagnosed according to criteria listed in the *Diagnostic and Statistical Manual of Mental Disorders*. Those criteria are:

> A. Recurrent episodes of binge eating. An episode of binge eating is characterized by both of the following:
> > (1) eating, in a discrete period of time (e.g., within any 2-hour period), an amount of food that is definitely larger than most people would eat during a similar period of time and under similar circumstances
> > (2) a sense of lack of control over eating during the episode (e.g., a feeling that one cannot stop eating or control what or how much one is eating)
> B. Recurrent inappropriate compensatory behavior in order to prevent weight gain, such as self-induced vomiting; misuse of laxatives, diuretics, enemas, or other medications; fasting; or excessive exercise.
> C. The binge eating and inappropriate compensatory behaviors both occur, on average, at least twice a week for three months.
> D. Self-evaluation is unduly influenced by body shape and weight.

Reprinted with permission from the Diagnostic and Statistical Manual of Mental Disorders, Fourth Edition, Text Revision. Copyright 2000 American Psychiatric Association.

E. The disturbance does not occur exclusively during episodes of anorexia nervosa.*

Bulimia is divided into two types:

Purging Type: during the current episode of bulimia nervosa, the person has regularly engaged in self-induced vomiting or the misuse of laxatives, diuretics, or enemas

Nonpurging Type: during the current episode of bulimia nervosa, the person has used other inappropriate compensatory behaviors, such as fasting or excessive exercise, but has not regularly engaged in self-induced vomiting or the misuse of laxatives, diuretics, or enemas*

Symptoms include:

• Weight gain or loss (though weight may be normal)
• Lethargy
• Bloating
• Swelling of the salivary glands (a result of the stimulation from binge eating and vomiting)
• Guilt, depression or anxiety
• Knuckle calluses or abrasions on hands
• Tooth enamel erosion or staining

Binges may be triggered by:

• Stress
• Depression
• Anxiety
• Disappointment

Complications include:

• Electrolyte imbalances that can lead to irregular heartbeats and even death
• Dental problems
• Rupture of the stomach or esophagus

*Reprinted with permission from the Diagnostic and Statistical Manual of Mental Disorders, Fourth Edition, Text Revision. Copyright 2000 American Psychiatric Association.

- Ulcers
- Chronic bowel problems and constipation

See the chapter on "Complications of Eating Disorders" for more information.

Bingeing is not the same as occasional overeating at a party or buffet. During a binge, a person may eat very large amounts of food much more rapidly than usual. There is a sense of loss of control during the binge. They often eat until they are uncomfortably full, and eat alone because of embarrassment about the amount of food consumed.

Binges happen in different ways for different people or even for one person. People have described going to several supermarkets to buy food for a single binge, so as not to arouse suspicion. Some go from restaurant to restaurant. Others have even resorted to stealing food. (Bingeing can be very expensive as well as embarrassing.)

The urge to binge is a natural consequence of restricting food. Any healthy individual who restricts food intake is at risk for bingeing.

CAROL'S STORY

Carol was an excellent student and a very good soccer player. She only wished she could be prettier. If she were thinner, she believed, she would be prettier. When she was thirteen years old, she saw a picture of herself and hated what she saw. That was the turning point for her. She felt that she had to do something, and her weight was something she thought she could control.

Carol started dieting, restricting calories just a little at first. As she lost weight, her diet became stricter. She was constantly hungry and became obsessed with thoughts of food, and soon began binge eating in secret, and then vomiting after binges to control her weight.

Both Carol's weight and her self-esteem were at an all-time low when she finally received the help she needed. Her basketball coach noticed that something was wrong and spoke to Carol's mother, who took her to her primary care physician. Even with good treatment, her recovery was slow and she was hospitalized several times, but slowly she began improving.

The struggle is not over, but Carol feels good about herself most of the time and she enjoys life. She takes pride in her schoolwork and is becoming more involved socially. Thinking back to the time when she was most ill, Carol says: "I was unapproachable and painfully thin. I was not a happy person. Even on bad days, I'll take now over then every time."

Binge-Eating Disorder

Binge-eating disorder is an eating disorder that, like the others, can have dangerous complications, and must be taken seriously. It is a relatively common disorder that affects both men and women. It occurs more often in adults than in teenagers and more often in women than in men. Binge-Eating Disorder (BED) was formerly known as compulsive overeating, but is now being recognized as an eating disorder, although it is still not formally classified as one.

People with binge-eating disorder have recurrent episodes of binge eating and often frequent failed attempts at trying to lose weight. They have a feeling of being out of control during the binge eating. Unlike people with bulimia, they do not have compensatory mechanisms such as self-induced vomiting to prevent weight gain.

About 50 percent of people with binge-eating disorder are overweight. People suffering from binge-eating disorder may use food to fill an emotional void, to hide from their emotions, or to cope with strong emotions and problems. As in the case of the other eating disorders, they almost always have low self-esteem. Like other eating disorders, BED is caused by a combination of psychological, physiological and socio-cultural factors.

The National Institute of Mental Health estimates that between 2 and 5 percent of Americans fit the criteria for binge–eating disorder in a 6-month period. It is present in about 8 percent of obese people and as many as 20 to 40 percent of obese people seeking treatment at weight-loss clinics. People usually begin binge eating in their late teens or twenties. About 40 percent of binge eating occurs in males.

The following may put one at increased risk for BED:

- Poor self-image
- Parental depression

- A significant bad childhood experience
- Exposure to negative comments about one's weight and shape
- Yo-yo dieting

Binge-eating disorder has not yet been formally classified as a specific eating disorder, so it falls into a category called "Eating Disorders Not Otherwise Specified." It will probably be formally classified as a specific eating disorder soon. Below you will find the research criteria or proposed criteria for diagnosing binge-eating disorder.

A. Recurrent episodes of binge eating. An episode of binge eating is characterized by both of the following:
>   (1) eating, in a discrete period of time (e.g., within any 2-hour period), an amount of food that is definitely larger than most people would eat in a similar period of time under similar circumstances
>   (2) a sense of lack of control over eating during the episode (e.g., a feeling that one cannot stop eating or control what or how much one is eating)

B. The binge-eating episodes are associated with three (or more) of the following:
>   (1) eating much more rapidly than normal
>   (2) eating until feeling uncomfortably full
>   (3) eating large amounts of food when not feeling physically hungry
>   (4) eating alone because of being embarrassed by how much one is eating
>   (5) feeling disgusted with oneself, depressed, or very guilty after overeating

C. Marked distress regarding binge eating is present

D. The binge eating occurs, on average, at least 2 days a week for 6 months....

E. The binge eating is not associated with the regular use of inappropriate compensatory behaviors (e.g., purging, fasting, excessive exercise) and does not occur exclusively during the course of Anorexia Nervosa or Bulimia Nervosa.*

---

*Reprinted with permission from the Diagnostic and Statistical Manual of Mental Disorders, Fourth Edition, Text Revision. Copyright 2000 American Psychiatric Association.

People often eat alone because of embarrassment about the amount of food eaten, and feel ashamed, depressed or guilty after the binge. Binges may be triggered by stress, depression, anxiety or disappointment, among other things.

For a doctor to diagnose binge-eating disorder, the binges must occur on average at least two days a week for six months, so a person who binges once or twice does not have binge-eating disorder. This is different from bulimia, because there is no regular use of behaviors such as vomiting, fasting, laxative or diuretic use, or excessive exercise.

Symptoms:

- Weight gain
- Large fluctuations in weight
- Eating large amounts of food when not hungry
- Feeling out of control when eating
- Buying excessive amounts of food or hiding food for a binge
- Lethargy
- Bloating
- Guilt and shame after overeating
- Depressed mood
- Low self-esteem

STEVEN'S STORY

Steven had a relatively happy, uneventful childhood. His mother had a mild depression that was well controlled on medication. The family was close and had many good times together.

As a child Steven was mildly overweight. He was an excellent student and enjoyed school for the most part, but does remember being teased about his weight on occasion. After graduating from high school, he left home to attend a competitive university, and over the course of the next year, he was involved in a number of difficult personal relationships.

Steven ate when he felt anxious, sad or stressed—particularly when he was stressed. He does not recall suddenly putting on a lot of weight. His weight just crept up gradually. Someone recommended a low-fat diet, which appealed to him. He followed this diligently for about 6 months, and lost a large amount of weight. He felt proud of his achievement, but was constantly hungry.

At a buffet lunch one day, he ate more than he was used to eating. He was guilty about "breaking" his diet, and skipped lunch the next day. By 4:00 that afternoon he was starving. He drove to a supermarket, stocked up on cookies, chips, and candies, and ate relentlessly. This set him up for a pattern of binge eating, which thereafter took place when he was hungry or stressed. By the end of the year, Steven had gained 40 pounds.

Eating Disorders Not Otherwise Specified

There are many other eating disorders or eating problems that don't quite meet the strict criteria of anorexia or bulimia. For example, if a woman with all the features of anorexia did not have amenorrhea (lack of menstrual periods), she would not be classified as having anorexia nervosa, and would fall into this "Eating Disorders Not Otherwise Specified" category. Another example would be someone who had fewer binge eating episodes per week than required for the strict diagnosis of bulimia. Someone who eats more than usual at times, without truly bingeing, and purges to lose weight would also have a "Not Specified" disorder. Binge-Eating Disorder, discussed above, also falls into this category, as it has not yet been formally classified as an eating disorder.

Nearly half of all patients with eating disorders presenting to eating disorder programs for treatment are diagnosed with "Eating Disorder Not Otherwise Specified." The diagnosis is especially common among teenagers. These eating disorders may not have specific names, but they are serious and need immediate treatment.

SARAH'S STORY

Sarah was seventeen years old when she was chosen to join a well-known dance group. In spite of the fact that she had never had a weight problem, she was always conscious about her body shape and her appearance in general. When she joined the group she noticed that most of the other dancers were thinner than she was. She began to feel self-conscious when rehearsing, especially around the time of menstruation, when she felt particularly "fat" and bloated. She was reassured by her mother that she was fine, and praised for her dancing skills, but this did not help Sarah's self-consciousness.

Sarah began dieting, and alternated this with episodes of eating more than usual. She also went to see a gynecologist for her symptoms of bloating before menstruation, and was prescribed a diuretic, to get rid of extra fluid. Using the diuretic made her feel temporarily less bloated on those days. When she had used up the medication, she called for a refill, which she was given. After that was used up, Sarah was embarrassed to call again, so she went to see a different physician for a prescription. This continued for a while, until Sarah's mother, noticing her weight fluctuating, took her to a physician specializing in eating disorders.

Sarah was one of the lucky ones, and is doing better with comprehensive treatment. Abusing diuretic medications or any other medication can lead to very serious health consequences. It is not a safe way to lose weight.

JANET'S STORY

Janet is an eighth grade honors student. Both her mother and sister are slightly overweight and she has watched them struggle with different diets. She herself had never had weight problems, but was always a little self-conscious of her body. She joined a dance group, in which she was urged to "drop a few pounds" to have a greater chance of being selected for bigger performances. She was embarrassed by the comment, but decided that she could afford to eat in a healthier way, so she began by cutting out red meats, and then all meats. She then cut out all candy and snacks. Although Janet does not have an eating disorder per se, positive reinforcement from her teacher on weight loss, combined with eating becoming more rigid, can put her at great risk.

COMPULSIVE EXERCISING—KATIE'S STORY

Katie's weight fluctuated between 100 pounds and 105 pounds. She was a college student and maintained her low weight by restricting her diet to mostly fruits and vegetables, and by exercising vigorously seven days a week. Keeping up with her school schedule, her studies, and her daily two hour exercise routine barely allowed Katie time to sleep. In spite of exhaustion, and back pain, she could not relax her exercise schedule. She remembers that on a day she spent on a trip with a group of students, she was anxious about being unable to exercise for one day; she felt ugly and fat.

Katie's story shows how compulsive exercising can occur as part of an eating disorder. It is not unusual for people with eating disorders to use excessive exercise as a form of weight control. They will sometimes exercise at great physical and psychological cost to themselves, and often feel extremely guilty if they are not able to exercise.

Just as other dangerous behaviors associated with eating disorders can put one at risk for serious complications, so can compulsive exercising. A person with anorexia nervosa and an already weakened heart can put him- or herself at increased risk with exercise. One can also be at increased risk for stress fractures and dehydration.

We all know that a moderate amount of exercise is good for us. Together with healthy eating, exercise can lower the risk of obesity, heart disease, diabetes, and high cholesterol. More than that, the right amount of exercise makes us feel good. Does that mean more exercise is better? Ideally most people who are healthy should exercise for at least 30 minutes on about five days per week. Some athletes may do significantly more than this. If the exercise remains enjoyable, and does not negatively affect them physically or mentally, this is usually not a problem.

However, some people with anorexia or bulimia may exercise compulsively, sometimes for several hours every day, to maintain a low weight. When they can't exercise they may feel fat, guilty, or even depressed. Exercise starts to interfere with their lives and their functioning. At this point exercise becomes harmful. Over-exercising can lead to back, leg or joint pain. Individuals with longstanding anorexia nervosa, who may have osteoporosis, are especially at risk. A person who doesn't eat enough calories will lose muscle mass despite exercising, and will increase his or her risk of injury.

In our society, just as dieting is often looked upon as "normal" behavior, so over-exercising is often accepted and even glorified. Magazines are filled with articles about fitness and the achievements of athletes. Their covers usually depict very thin women or muscular men. Companies are making millions of dollars on fitness equipment which may or may not work. Young men and women often feel that they don't "measure up," and are joining health clubs in droves to try to achieve their ideal body image. The message gets confused. Yes, exercise is a good thing, and yes, too much exercise is harmful. Apart from the negative physical effects of too much exercise, the psychological effects can be harmful. Trying to be healthy and toned is a good thing, but when the focus on weight, shape, and exercise consumes one's life, and one's self-image becomes tied to the way one looks, a problem exists. Remember that compulsive exercise may be part of an eating disorder.

Who is at risk for compulsive exercising?

- People with eating disorders
- Athletes
- Men and women with low self-esteem

Warning signs that you may be exercising too much:

- You exercise more than once a day.
- You exercise to change your weight or appearance, rather than to become fit.
- You no longer enjoy your workout.
- You often exercise rather than study or socialize.
- You insist on exercising even under very difficult circumstances.
- You exercise in spite of injury.
- You exercise against medical advice.
- You become very anxious or depressed if unable to exercise for a day.
- Your self-image is strongly related to your exercise achievements.

BODY DYSMORPHIC DISORDER

Body dysmorphic disorder affects both men and women. It is a condition in which people have a preoccupation about an imagined or insignificant defect in their appearance. The preoccupation can involve any part of the body, but areas of the head and face are most commonly involved. All patients are affected to some degree, but some become severely impaired. The disorder affects their social life and their work. Some even become housebound. People with body dysmorphic disorder often have low self-esteem, and may suffer from severe depression.

An effective treatment for body dysmorphic disorder seems to be cognitive behavioral therapy, a form of psychotherapy. Medications such as antidepressants may be useful too.

Body dysmorphic disorder will be more fully discussed later in the book in the chapter on "Body Image and Self-Esteem."

MUSCLE DYSMORPHIA

Reverse anorexia or muscle dysmorphia is probably a form of body dysmorphic disorder. It can occur in either sex but is much more common in men. The person has a distorted body image and feels as if he is small and puny in spite of the fact that he is often quite large. In spite of having large muscles, a person with muscle dysmorphia is preoccupied with the fact that his muscles are too small. He may abuse anabolic steroids or spend excessive time at the gym, to the point of endangering his health.

What Are Your Food and Body Image Concerns?

Many teenagers don't have full-blown eating disorders, but still have food and body image concerns. Do you recognize some of these symptoms in yourself? If you do, it is probably worth asking for help.

- Being overly concerned about your body weight or shape
- Feeling embarrassed about eating in front of people
- Having frequent thoughts about food and calories
- Eating in an out of control manner
- Frequently eating when you are not hungry
- Dieting or skipping meals
- Weighing yourself frequently
- Food rituals, such as cutting food up into tiny pieces
- Seeing yourself as fat even when others say you are thin
- Believing that your value as a person is tied in to the way you look and how much you weigh

It is rare for a young person not to be concerned about his or her body at some time or another. Sometimes it may be difficult to decide if you are accurately assessing your size or health.

If you have decided that you would like to become thinner or fitter:

• Start by speaking to your parents about your desire to become thinner or fitter.

• Get checked by your primary care doctor to see if you are in the normal weight range and whether or not it would be safe to lose weight. By using objective measures like the growth chart and your body mass index, doctors really do know what you should weigh to be in the healthy range.

• Speak to your doctor or a nutritionist about your goals; have these professionals help you form a healthy nutrition and exercise plan. Make sure that you are getting enough calories and fats to grow and develop healthily. The teenage years are an important time for growth.

• Ask your family to be involved in healthy lifestyle changes. You could take walks or plan healthy recipes together.

• Because this is a time when you may still be growing, it is always important to be monitored regularly. Make sure that you are eating balanced meals and that your weight remains in the safe range.

In summary, eating disorders and their related conditions can manifest in a number of ways and at different ages, but they should always be taken seriously. If you are struggling with an eating disorder, know that you are not alone. There is help available. Understanding that they can occur in both males and females, in any age or cultural group, and recognizing their early warning signs, can go a long way toward preventing much of the suffering that is too common among people with chronic eating disorders.

3

Who Develops an
Eating Disorder and Why?

We now know that eating disorders do not only occur in teenage girls from wealthy families in Western cultures. They affect males and females of all ages from various backgrounds and cultures. Although it's true that most people with eating disorders first develop this condition when they are adolescents, eating disorders can occur in children as young as 6 or 7 and in adults as old as 60 or 70. Sadly, more than 50 percent of teenagers are unhappy with their bodies, and those who measure their self-worth by the way they look, and have a negative body image, are at increased risk for an eating disorder.

Although women are diagnosed with eating disorders much more often than are men, we now believe that eating disorders are more common in men than was previously believed. For a number of reasons, boys and men do not seek treatment as often and are not diagnosed as early. They may be embarrassed about having an illness that was in the past thought to be a "female problem." There are also not many eating disorder centers treating males, and because they may not think of it, health care providers may miss the diagnosis in men even when their illness brings them to a doctor's office. For all these reasons it is difficult to estimate the true incidence in boys and men, but it is thought to be about 10 percent of total cases.

About 8 million Americans suffer from eating disorders. The

National Institute of Mental Health estimates that in females the lifetime risk for anorexia is between 0.5 and 3.7 percent, and for bulimia is between 1.1 and 4.2 percent, although the incidence of bulimia is much higher in certain groups such as college-aged women. Although the prevalence of eating disorders among adults seems constant, the prevalence among teenagers appears to have increased. Maybe this is partly due to increased awareness and earlier diagnosis. Maybe it is due to increased advertising and media pressure directed at younger and younger people.

What Causes an Eating Disorder?

There is no one cause for eating disorders. Personality traits, family and environmental factors, and cultural influences all play a role. Certain combinations of these factors can lead a susceptible person to develop an eating disorder. For that susceptible person, all it may take is a well-intentioned comment from someone, such as "It looks like you gained a little weight," or even "You look better. You are not as skinny as you were," to tip him or her over the edge. Eating disorders, which were once rare outside of Western culture, are spreading from America to other continents. Japan, China and Spain, among others, have seen an increase in eating disorders as they adopt many of the Western values. I have also interviewed young women from Israel, where eating disorders seem to be increasing. These countries need to be studied further to determine the size of the problem.

DIETING

A common underlying feature in the development of an eating disorder is dieting. Americans spend billions of dollars per year to lose weight on diets and products that usually don't even work. Advertising companies are very interested in marketing to teenagers. At any one time, about two-thirds of teenage girls are dieting. Although by no means does everyone who goes on a diet develop a problem, most eating disorders will begin with a diet. People who go on a restrictive diet for a significant period of time develop hunger and obsessions about food, which puts them at risk for either excessive dieting or binge eating.

Our Relationship with Food

We eat food for balanced nutrition, but we also eat for pleasure (because food tastes good), for social reasons, and for comfort in times of stress. Food and emotions are strongly connected, and for some people the relationship with food goes wrong. Instead of being seen as nutritional and satisfying, food becomes a forbidden temptation or something feared. This results in abnormal eating or a full-blown eating disorder.

Today more food choices are available than ever before, but many of these choices involve foods that are highly processed, often with high fat and sugar contents. Another possible problem with food in today's society is that the family often does not sit down to a meal together. Teenagers are especially likely to eat on the go. They may eat at fast-food restaurants, binge, or skip meals completely. If they are away at college, there may be minimal supervision, and eating may become more erratic. These bad habits may trigger an eating disorder in a susceptible person.

Genetics and Biological Factors

There appears to be a strong genetic predisposition to anorexia and bulimia, as was shown in family and twin studies. Although cultural factors play an important role, most people exposed to these cultural factors do not develop eating disorders. This fact leads researchers to believe that certain people may be genetically at higher risk. An imbalance of neurotransmitters, including serotonin, has also been thought to contribute to an eating disorder. It is possible that medications affecting these neurotransmitters may play a role in treatment.

Personality

People with anorexia can often be introverted, perfectionistic and sensitive to criticism. They frequently have obsessive-compulsive tendencies, or are prone to anxiety. They sometimes have a strong desire to please others and are afraid of conflict or "rocking the boat." They are often dependent on others for approval. Parents often describe them as good, compliant or "perfect" children. Of course, not everyone with anorexia nervosa fits this category.

People with bulimia are often more extroverted, dramatic and impulsive. They are also able to enjoy things. Some may have a history of being overweight and being exposed to criticism about their weight. Some people with bulimia abuse drugs or alcohol.

People who develop binge-eating disorder also may have been exposed to negative comments about their weight and shape.

LOW SELF-ESTEEM

A common trait in people with eating disorders is low self-esteem. During adolescence, girls become acutely aware of their bodies, how they compare to others, and how they believe others perceive them. A mother's attitude toward her daughter's body has a big influence on that daughter's attitude toward her own body and therefore an influence on her body image, and ultimately, her self-esteem. Some girls feel they don't measure up to others, and their solution may be to start dieting. In certain situations, this dieting can be the beginning of an eating disorder.

DEPRESSION

People with eating disorders may have a history of depression. Also, in a person who has difficulty with separation, the period of having to move from home to college can be stressful enough to trigger a problem. The teenage girl with anorexia, for example, may also have difficulty with the transition to adulthood and the physical changes that are associated with this. Losing weight can be a way to delay sexual maturation. Teenagers with anorexia nervosa have small hips and very little breast tissue and do not menstruate. Anorexia may be a silent protest against growing up—a way to remain a child. An eating disorder may also be the way she copes with life, depression and personal or family problems. The problems of life and growing up can feel so overwhelming. The eating disorder gives her one thing to worry about, one thing to obsess about. It may be the only way she feels in control. A young girl told me, as she was recovering, that her biggest fear was getting well. When she could no longer obsess about food and weight, she would have to deal with other issues. How would she deal with everything going on around her and in the world? How would she relate to friends and boyfriends? How would she cope with life?

FAMILY

Problems and conflict in the family can either be a cause or a result of an eating disorder. When someone in the family has an eating disorder, it affects all the other family members in some way. Some causes of stress in the family include divorce or separation, loss of a job, alcoholism, or even a new birth. The eating disorder and the constant obsession with food and weight can be seen as a way to escape from these other problems, or a way to take the focus off them.

It's not useful to place blame on a family, because usually it is a number of causes that have led to the eating disorder, and most families have tried to do the very best they can. Blaming the family can interfere with the family support and involvement that is often so important in helping someone recover from an eating disorder. Also, focusing blame in one direction or another takes away energy needed to get well.

The following problems, however, may be found in families of patients with eating disorders.

• Families may tend to be perfectionistic, and may be more critical. Some children model this "perfect" behavior, and others feel they will never live up to the expectations, so they give up. Some develop an eating disorder.

• There may be a family member with depression.

• Families may have more conflict, and may have difficulty resolving conflict.

• There may be parental pressure to lose weight. A parent may have a history of an eating disorder or obesity.

• There may be a history of criticism regarding weight.

• Family members may be too dependent on each other.

• There may be poor communication in the family. In some families, the only effective way to communicate is without words. Refusing to eat and losing weight may be a way of saying something that cannot be said in words.

FRIENDS

Sometimes a person's friends increase the risk of dieting behavior and possibly an eating disorder. Friends who are interested in dieting and achieving a thin ideal; friends who are engaging in bingeing or purging behaviors; and being teased by friends can all trigger eating disorders in a susceptible person.

CULTURAL FACTORS

Eating disorders occur in all cultures and all socio-economic groups. At present, however, they are more common in developed countries and more affluent cultures with Western values—partly because being thin is more valued in Western cultures. It is almost impossible to live in the United States without being constantly bombarded with messages about looking better and becoming thinner. Female models and actresses have become noticeably thinner over the years. Think back to a past beauty ideal, Marilyn Monroe. She would have been considered overweight by today's model standards. On television, in magazines, in movies and now on the internet, you will see images of often unattainably thin women, and hear about the latest diet fads. Many young girls try to look like the very thin supermodels of today. Unfortunately, to do so, they usually have to severely restrict calories, live with obsessions about food and weight, and suffer serious medical and mental consequences. Sadly, they are less likely to achieve their ideal than they are to develop an eating disorder.

Think about it: The businesses that feature those super-thin models make a lot of money by making us strive for a perfection that never can be achieved!

Keep in mind that those models are not a healthy ideal. Several of them have even spoken out about the health risks they took in order to lose weight. It is very possible that many have eating disorders themselves.

And just how "real" are the models in those photographs, anyway? They have clothiers, make-up artists and personal hairdressers working on them for hours. Lighting changes the way they look in the pictures, and advertising photographs are airbrushed to give the illusion of perfect bodies.

Don't buy these ideas of the way you should look.

In some cases, eating disorders are glorified. The word thin is sometimes used interchangeably with the word anorexic, and some young women actually appreciate being told that they look "anorexic." Young women are receiving the message that being thin makes them beautiful and successful. At the same time we live in a time when we have an excess of food available, and we are also being urged to buy these foods. And don't forget, people enjoy eating good foods! Young people are getting mixed messages. No wonder they are confused.

I pulled several magazines aimed at women off the shelf. Almost every cover had an article about losing weight or looking more beautiful. These were some of their cover messages.

"Lose 20 lbs. by June."—*Good Housekeeping*, May 2002.

"Fighting weight. Stars talk about their struggles."—*Us Weekly*, November 2001.

"Getting Gorgeous! Stars share their secret tips and tricks."—*In Style*, April 2002.

Everywhere we turn, we see messages like these, and unfortunately young girls and women are led to believe that being thin and beautiful is of utmost importance.

Media messages are not only aimed at women. Today, male models are leaner and much more muscular, and even young boys are being targeted, with new bigger, more muscular action figures—again, with bodies that are impossible to achieve.

CHRONIC ILLNESS

People with certain chronic illnesses such as diabetes mellitus are at increased risk for the development of eating disorders. One reason is that the chronic illness may contribute to low self-esteem. Also, from early on people with diabetes are taught to monitor their diets and blood sugars closely. In some people this can lead to an obsession about calorie intake, diet and weight, which can set them up for the development of an eating disorder. Another reason may be that patients with type 2 diabetes often experience some weight loss at the onset, and then gain weight after starting insulin. Some patients may withhold their insulin in order to lose weight. This is an extremely dangerous practice and can cause serious complications of diabetes including death.

STRESSFUL LIFE EVENTS

The onset of an eating disorder often follows some stressful life event, which may or may not be catastrophic. Physical or mental illness, such as depression, separation from a loved one, or a history of sexual abuse may precipitate an eating disorder.

Examples of possible stresses include leaving home for college; losing a friend or partner; family problems; divorce; and family illness.

Another significant stress is sexual abuse. There seems to be a higher incidence of sexual abuse among people with eating disorders. Researchers have several theories about why this might be so. Perhaps patients develop an eating disorder in order to regain control over their bodies. Or perhaps the eating disorder serves as a way to protect them by making them less physically attractive and less sexual. It's important to know, however, that not everyone who is sexually abused develops an eating disorder, and by no means has everyone with an eating disorder been sexually abused.

Eating Disorders Among Athletes

For a number of reasons athletes are at increased risk for disordered eating, dangerous weight loss methods, over-exercising and eating disorders.

An acquaintance of mine enrolled her thirteen-year-old son in wrestling. He was required to lose ten pounds by any means as quickly as possible to "make weight" for the team. At least one member of the team fainted because of dieting and restricting fluids. My friend's son restricted his food intake and resorted to "sweating" himself on the day of the weigh-in to lose more water weight. He reached his target, and then began bingeing on all those foods of which he had been deprived. His weight yo-yoed up and down for years.

Why do people participate in sports? There are many reasons, including enjoyment and socialization. They may take part to relieve stress, or because they like competition and challenge. Some people participate in sports for health reasons, including an effort to change body weight or shape.

The athlete with an eating disorder uses exercise predominantly as a means of controlling his or her weight or shape.

There are several possible reasons why athletes and dancers are at risk for eating disorders. They may feel increased pressure to become thin for aesthetic appeal or for enhanced performance. Also, some of their personality traits, which include perfectionism, being competitive, and being extremely focused on their achievement in a specific area, match those of people with eating disorders. (There are important differences too, particularly the fact that athletes do not typically have low self-esteem.) They may have an intense desire to please others. Finally, athletes are often at their peak when they are teenagers or young adults, which is also the time that eating disorders often present.

Sports and activities that require a low body weight can put both men and women at risk for developing eating disorders. These activities include wrestling, modeling, track, ballet and gymnastics, among others. The 2002 Winter Olympics brought this problem to light as it related to ski-jumpers. The ski-jumpers, in order to gain a competitive edge, often keep a low-calorie, low-fat diet, which results in a low body fat percentage. There is concern that this condition, sometimes known as "anorexia athletica," can put someone at risk for developing full-blown anorexia nervosa with all its complications. (*The Washington Post*, Feb. 19, 2002, Liz Clarke.)

Sometimes, athletes who injure themselves may begin to eat abnormally. Because of the fear of weight gain while not exercising, they may drastically restrict their food intake.

We are gradually learning about the dangers of eating disorders and their prevalence amongst athletes. It's important for athletes and coaches to be aware of their harmful effects both on health and ultimately on athletic performance.

How Much Exercise Is Too Much?

That's hard to say. What is considered excessive exercise for some people may not be excessive for an athlete. We have found that it is not the amount of exercise as much as it is the attitudes toward exercise that determines whether there is a problem.

• Usually a person exercises to increase fitness, but athletes with eating disorders may exercise solely for weight loss or to affect their appearance. Their self-image and self-esteem are tied to their exercising and their appearance.

• The athlete with an eating disorder may exercise with excessive intensity even in the face of an injury.

• The athlete with an eating disorder is often very rigid with his or her exercise schedule, and may be very distressed about missing a workout. That athlete may even miss important meetings or social activities to prevent missing a workout.

Patients with eating disorders who exercise excessively are putting themselves at risk both physically and mentally.

FEMALE ATHLETIC TRIAD

Female athletes are at increased risk for the development of eating disorders. One reason is that they believe (wrongly) that losing weight and body fat will improve their performance. What happens instead is that they lose muscle and in severe cases even heart muscle, and eventually health and performance both suffer.

A condition that we find in certain female athletes with disordered eating is known as the athletic triad.

The key symptoms are:

• Disordered eating
• Loss of menstrual periods
• Osteoporosis (thinning of the bones)

These symptoms are caused by these very active girls getting inadequate nutrition and fats, which in turn causes them to have low levels of estrogen and to stop menstruating. This triad may affect girls who participate in gymnastics, long-distance running, or ballet. Cheerleaders, swimmers, and divers, who may also have a drive for thinness, are also at risk. To keep their weight down, they may diet, vomit, or use pills. Some develop eating disorders. Low weight and excessive exercise may delay puberty. Girls who have begun to menstruate may stop. This can result in osteoporosis.

BRENDA'S STORY

For Brenda, it was a combination of events that triggered her eating disorder. Her best friend had moved away the previous year, and Brenda had recently moved to a new school where she found it difficult to make new friends. She felt lonely, and thought that she would be accepted if she became fitter and thinner. She began dieting and exercising obsessively. Although Brenda received some compliments about her weight loss at first, rather than become more popular, she became more and more isolated and withdrawn.

The Effects of Food Restriction

During the Second World War, Dr. Ancel Keys and his colleagues closely observed a group of male volunteers to evaluate the effects of starvation. These were healthy men who willingly entered this study. Their food intake was severely restricted for a number of months, and they were closely monitored with respect to health and psychological status. Interesting findings emerged from this distressing study. The men, being deprived of nutrition, began developing many of the behaviors (including obsessions about food and food preparation) seen in typical anorexic patients. Once they resumed eating, a number of the men developed binge eating behaviors or other eating disturbances. This study taught us a lot about the symptoms and physiology of anorexia nervosa, and let us understand that many of the symptoms can be caused by starvation itself.

What Keeps Eating Disorders Going?

As I have discussed, certain conditions trigger eating disorders in susceptible people, and then there are perpetuating factors that keep the disorders going. In the case of anorexia nervosa, frequent compliments on weight loss initially can be a strong motivating factor to keep dieting. The biological effects of starvation can be a stimulant, and some people have described the feelings of a "high." Also, the eating disorder provides an identity for the anorexic patient who might otherwise be struggling to find one. An example is someone graduating from high school. She may be insecure and unsure of her plans for the future. The eating disorder may give her an identity and a sense of achievement. The eating disorder can be her way of coping. During treatment, these issues are considered, because for someone to get well, the unhealthy identity and goals need to be replaced with healthier ones.

In the case of bulimia or binge-eating disorder, the first binge may be all about food, but eventually the cycle becomes a way of regulating mood and of coping. It becomes a way of dealing with anxiety, fear, depression and loneliness.

Some reasons why people binge and purge

- To cope with stress.
- To cope with anxiety.
- To deal with disappointment.
- To avoid dealing with feelings.

Almost anything can trigger a binge, but the people I spoke to mentioned the following:

- Feeling very hungry
- Being alone
- Feeling depressed
- Feeling fat
- Feeling anxious
- Eating out

Don't forget that bingeing is a habit, and like any habit, can be hard to break.

Summary of Some of the Risk Factors for Developing an Eating Disorder

- Low self-esteem.
- Dieting.

- Feelings of lack of control.
- History of being teased.
- History of comments about needing to lose weight, by someone of influence, e.g. coach, dance instructor.
- Participation in sports or activities requiring low weight or increased musculature.
- Personal or family history of obesity.
- Personal or family history of depression.
- Family history of an eating disorder.
- Gay orientation in males.
- History of abuse.
- History of family conflict or excessive parental expectation.
- Culture which places high value on external appearance or thinness. (Note: Teenage girls in our culture are at increased risk.)

Could you have an eating disorder?

If you answer yes to one or more of the following questions, it may be worth checking with your physician.

1. Do you worry about your weight frequently?
2. Do you spend a lot of time thinking about food, fat and calories?
3. Have you lost weight?
4. Does your weight fluctuate significantly?
5. Are you dieting?
6. Do you feel out of control when eating?
7. Do you throw up after eating?
8. Do you use any pills or medications to lose weight?
9. Do you exercise excessively?
10. Does the way you feel about yourself depend on how you look or how much you weigh?

If you still have questions about whether you, or a friend or family member, may have an eating disorder, see Chapter 6, "Warning Signs of an Eating Disorder."

4

Body Image and Self-Esteem

For she who only finds her self-esteem
In other's admiration, begs in alms;
Depends on others for her daily food,
And is the very servant of her slaves....
—Joanna Baillie (1762–1851),
"The Countess of Albini"

This quotation is more than 200 years old, but it is still relevant today. It emphasizes just how dependent we can become on what other people think of us. Instead of basing self-esteem on character, accomplishments, and real self-worth, sadly, some people depend mainly on others for approval.

Body Image

Body image is the way we feel about our bodies and how we look. For some people, body image is closely tied into how they feel about themselves and their lives in general. People who feel very unhappy about how they look, or feel they could only have a happy life if they were thinner or taller or prettier, for example, have a negative body image. These people believe that their value and self-worth is measured by how they look, rather than what they stand for and what they have accomplished. When they feel out of control, some people may try to gain control by controlling their bodies and their weight. Ironically, instead of achieving control, their abnormal psychological drive for thinness combined with their altered perception of their bodies, leads to loss of control over their bodies, their weight and their lives.

What influences your body image? There are many possibilities:

- Family
- Friends
- Influential people such as coaches or dance teachers
- Culture
- Media

The beauty industries are constantly trying to make people buy products to make them look more perfect. Millions of dollars are spent on diet supplements, cosmetics, exercise equipment, and plastic surgery, all supposedly to help people achieve a sometimes impossible ideal.

One young woman told me that she was strongly influenced by watching a popular sit-com with three pretty but very thin actresses. It's important for teenagers to recognize that many of the images of models and actresses we look up to are not real. Actresses often have make-up artists and hairdressers at hand. The photographs of models who grace magazine covers are often airbrushed to minimize their imperfections. Nobody is perfect, and if you are struggling to reach perfection, you are setting yourself up for a lifelong battle. We may all be imperfect, but the positive side is that each of us is unique, with wonderful qualities. Spend some time thinking about your good points, and concentrate on those qualities that make you special.

A well-known model has revealed information about her history and the modeling industry. She spoke openly about her struggles to maintain a size 4 figure, and how she starved herself and even resorted to the use of drugs. She almost lost her life before she decided to make a change. She now accepts her average-size body and continues to be very successful in her field.

How Does a Negative Body Image Develop?

Teasing is one thing that can lead to a negative body image. Being exposed to teasing or criticism about one's looks or weight at a young age can put a person at increased risk for poor body image and an eating disorder. One young woman who has an older, slender sister said she could never forget being labeled as "the chubby one" as she was growing up. Another told me that her dieting and eating disorder began when her dance instructor remarked that she would be a great dancer if she lost a few pounds.

Criticism is another powerful influence. Repeated negative remarks about appearance, even from one parent to another, may have an affect on a child's body image.

Prejudice in our society against people who are obese is another factor in negative body image, as is media endorsement of certain body ideals for men and women.

Occasional negative thoughts about one's body are not unusual, but when these bad thoughts dominate a person's life, that person has a negative body image. Teenagers, because they are already dealing with many physical and emotional changes, are especially vulnerable. A negative body image can stand in the way of accomplishments. It can also lead to depression and poor eating habits. Someone with a negative body image and low self-esteem who begins a diet is especially at risk for developing an eating disorder.

On the bright side, *positive* self-esteem messages from family and friends can help promote a positive body image. Good messages are those that promote accepting someone for who they are and not for the way they lock.

Remember: Beauty Ideals Change

It's interesting to keep in mind, as many Americans strive to achieve a thin ideal, that beauty ideals change and have changed over the years, and also that beauty ideals differ greatly across cultures.

In centuries past, even in Western cultures, being overweight was very acceptable, even desirable. It signified abundance and wealth. The people depicted in old paintings were often round and full-figured. Today, models and pageant contestants are significantly thinner than they were only a few decades ago. If we asked our grandparents what their beauty ideal was when they were teenagers, it would be very different from ours today. The American beauty ideal changed dramatically in the 1960s with the rise in fame of the super-thin model Twiggy. Today our beauty ideals are often unhealthy.

Beauty ideals differ tremendously across cultures even today, although it is true that certain cultures are adopting Western values. In certain parts of Africa and parts of the Middle East, for example, an ideal body for women would be round and full, rather than very thin.

Not only do beauty ideals change over the years, they change with the beholder. One person's idea of beauty may be different from another's.

However we may perceive external beauty, we must remember that it does not last. Meanwhile, true beauty is much more than what we see on the outside. A combination of things, including good character, makes one beautiful inside. This type of beauty can last forever.

Self-esteem

Having a good body image is only part of what makes up good self-esteem. Self-esteem means liking yourself inside and out. Positive self-esteem means that you don't rely on others for approval. It shields you from insensitive remarks. It can give you courage, and help you through difficult times and disappointments.

ROBERT'S STORY

In high school Robert was one of the smartest boys I knew. He didn't spend much time with friends, because he was always studying. His clothes were outdated, because he really didn't care for fashion trends. However, even though he hardly socialized, he was always willing to help students solve their complicated math or science problems, or lend a helping hand with English or Latin. Robert was teased, in part because he just didn't fit in, and in part because the people who teased him were jealous. He was well aware that behind his back he was known as a geek, but this didn't bother him a bit. He worked hard and was proud of his accomplishments, and comfortable with who he was. Robert had high self-esteem.

Body Image Study

I was interested in looking at the incidence of dieting and body dissatisfaction in a university setting and finding out the extent to which male and female university students differed with respect to their body image. I therefore designed a questionnaire and had copies given randomly to 100 students between the ages of eighteen and twenty-seven at a large East Coast university. The questions related to issues such as how they felt about their bodies and their weight, what had influenced their body image, and whether they had ever dieted. Their answers were very interesting, and pointed out some of the differences between those men and women when it came to dieting practices and feeling comfortable with the way they look.

You will find a copy of the questionnaire at the end of the chapter. Consider answering the questionnaire yourself to see how you rate. The scoring system will be explained below.

Forty-two students responded to the study. Of these, 27 were female and 15 were male. Eighteen of the females were unhappy or had mixed feelings about their body weight or shape, and of these, 11 had been teased. Of the nine who were happy about their weight and shape, only four had been teased. Fifteen of the 27 women had dieted, and the youngest reported age of first dieting was 10 years. Of the 15 who had dieted, 12 were unhappy or had mixed feelings about their body or weight, and 11 had been teased. Of the 12 who had never dieted, four had been teased.

The women rated the most important influences on their ideal body image as being the media and the mirror (equally). They cited the events that triggered their first diets as teasing, clothes not fitting, and a dance instructor recommending weight loss. All but two said they worried about their weight or shape at least sometimes, and six worried daily, but 22 of the 27 said that appearance did not affect their judgment of others.

Five of the 15 males who responded were unhappy or had mixed feelings about their bodies, and of these five, four had been teased. Three had dieted, and of those, two had been teased. The youngest age at first diet was 11 years. For the question "What has been the most important influence on your ideal body image," most men marked the category labeled "other," noting specific influences such as sports. The next most common answers were media, mirror and friends equally. The only event reported as triggering a first diet was having to make weight for Little League football. Ten said they worried about their weight and shape sometimes, two often, and three never. None reported worrying daily. Eleven of the 15 said that appearance did not affect their judgment of others.

I asked the females what, if anything, they would want to change about their appearance. Most of them reported wanting to change their lower bodies, i.e., their thighs, bottoms, "stomachs" (abdomens) and hips. Almost every male that wished to change something about his body reported wanting to have larger muscles, become taller or have stronger arms.

Body Image Questionnaire

1. What is your age? _____ years
2. What is your sex? Female _____ Male _____
3. What has been the most important influence on your ideal body image?

    Rank in order, number 1 being most important.
    Parents _____
    Friends _____
    Media: TV, magazines _____
    Photographs of yourself _____
    The mirror _____
    Other _____
4. Are you happy with your body weight and shape?

    Yes _____ No _____ Uncertain/Mixed feelings _____
5. Have you ever been teased about your body or weight?

    Yes _____ No _____

6. Have you ever dieted? Yes _____ No _____
7. If yes, at what age did you first diet?
8. If anything, what would you want to change about your body? List up to 3 things: _____
9. Did a certain event trigger your first diet? Yes _____ No _____
   If so, what? _____
10. Do you worry about your weight and shape
    Never _____
    Sometimes _____
    Often _____
    Daily _____
11. Do you think you will ever achieve your ideal body image?
    Yes _____ No _____
12. Check which you would rather have happen:
    Losing 10 pounds this year _____ Ranking in the top 10 of your class _____
13. Do you eat 3 meals a day?
    Most of the time _____
    Sometimes _____
    Almost never _____
14. Do you exercise for 45 minutes or longer:
    6 times/week or more _____
    Between 3 and 6 times / week _____
    2 time /week or less _____
15. How do you view others who are overweight?
    Positively _____ Negatively _____
    Neither. Appearance does not affect your judgment of others _____

Calculating your score:

Scores will be assigned only to numbers 4 through 6, and numbers 10 through 13.

Number 4: If you answered yes, give yourself 0; for uncertain, 1; and for no, 2.

Number 5: For yes 1, for no 0.

Number 6: For yes 1, for no 0.

Number 10: For never 0, for sometimes 1, for often 2, and for daily 3.

Number 11: For yes 0, and for no 1.

Number 12: For losing 10 pounds 1, and for ranking in the top 10, 0.

Number 13: For most of the time 0, and for sometimes or almost never 1.

Scores range from 0 to 10. If you scored less than 5, you are at lower risk for (less likely to have) a poor body image. If you scored 5 or more, you are at greater risk for (more likely to have) a poor body image. Note that the study and questionnaire are informal, and not necessarily scientific or conclusive, as the results are based on a small sample.

5

Eating Disorders in Males

All of the eating disorders discussed earlier can occur in males as well as in females. Their symptoms are similar in males, but there are subtle differences in the underlying causes and precipitating factors. Treatment outcomes are also similar, but parts of treatment may have to be modified for males.

Sadly, eating disorders in males are often not recognized, and even when they are, limited resources still exist for them.

Some Typical Cases

MAX'S STORY

Max began dieting at the age of 16. When he was a young boy his parents always considered him to be a little overweight, but he was quite comfortable with the way he looked until he entered the ninth grade and tried out for athletics. A friend on the team made an insensitive comment, saying Max was too heavy to make it round the track. Max tried to shrug off the remark, but he remembers the pain he felt to this day. Now 18 years old, when he looks at old pictures he says that he really wasn't fat, but he remembers that he certainly felt fatter and less fit than anyone else. He made up his mind that he was going to lose weight, and prove that he could make it round that field as fast as anyone else could.

He began by skipping school lunches. His parents didn't notice anything at first, as lunches were provided at school. He then started eating less for dinner, and after a month it became obvious that he was losing weight. His family and friends complimented him, assuming that his weight loss was caused by his busy schedule and his newly active life. The possibility of an eating disorder couldn't have been further from their minds. After all, he was a boy, and eating disorders were considered to be unusual among boys.

By the time Max had lost 18 pounds, he seemed to be a different person—but not in a good way. Not only did he look different, but he no longer enjoyed socializing, and he spent a whole lot of time alone in his room. He was hungry most of the day, and began obsessing about foods, foods he had not tasted for so long. He spent lunchtime alone, either reading or walking in the school grounds. He began to feel lonely and depressed.

One night Max came home late after a basketball game. He felt weaker than usual, as it was past his usual dinnertime. His parents had left dinner out for him, havng eaten earlier and gone out to an evening function. Max was alone at home and ravenous. All he had eaten that day was an apple for breakfast and a granola bar before the game. He looked over at the chicken and rice his mom had cooked, and then glanced at the chocolate cake in the fridge. No one else was there. He quickly ate the chicken and rice, but he didn't feel quite satisfied. He cut a sliver of chocolate cake, something he hadn't had for months. The taste was unbelievable. He cut one more slice neatly, hoping that no one would notice that any cake was missing. He was no longer hungry, but he craved something else. He searched through the cupboards and found two boxes of old Girl Scout cookies. He finished them. He now felt sick and disgusted with himself, and went to sleep, not wanting to think.

The following morning, remembering what he had done, and devastated by the belief that he had undone all his hard work, he decided that he would skip breakfast and lunch. He came home from school at 4:00, weak and dizzy. He had dinner with the family and then made an excuse that he had lots of studying to do. As soon as his parents had gone to bed, he crept into the kitchen and looked for anything he could eat: a box of crackers and cheese, old Halloween candy, and the remaining chocolate cake. Again he went to sleep, full and disgusted.

Max continued this pattern for several weeks, bingeing at night and restricting foods by day, and becoming more sad and withdrawn. Max had heard of people who made themselves throw up after eating, and he did try on several occasions, but he could never throw up. By this time his athletics coach had noticed that something was seriously wrong. He knew that Max wasn't eating lunch, and his teammates had complained that he avoided them. The coach spoke to his parents, who took him to a physician. The physician confirmed the eating disorder. Max entered treatment, and gradually he resumed a more regular pattern of eating.

Now he no longer feels hungry all day and no longer binge-eats at night. Because he has more energy he is able to exercise regularly and has not had a problem with his weight. Max was lucky that someone was able to recognize his eating disorder at an early stage and get him the treatment he needed. Unfortunately, sometimes eating disorders can go unrecognized for long periods of time—until serious medical and psychological complications have resulted.

DAVE'S STORY

Dave is 19 years old and has been struggling with body image and eating issues since the age of 17, when he left home to attend college. His problem went unrecognized until recently, when he was finally able to talk to his parents and his doctor about his illness. He had never been overweight, but neither had he conformed to the desired "male standard" in high school. He was neither tall nor muscular. Instead, he was smaller than most of his friends, and was not very competitive. He wasn't really interested in sports, and was never among the first few to be chosen for the athletic teams. Often he was the object of merciless teasing, and over the years his body image and self-esteem reached an all-time low.

Soon after he began college, his parents separated. This loss, combined with leaving home, and his having a poor self-image, caused Dave to become withdrawn from his friends. He had always been very aware of his appearance, and even as a child used to wish he could be fitter and leaner. Being away from home, he decided that he could have more control over his eating and his body.

The college cafeteria offered mostly high-fat foods and non-nutritious snacks. He ate these sparingly and survived on apples and oranges between meals. After classes, instead of going out with his friends, he worked out at the college gym. Dave started losing weight, but instead of feeling better about himself, he felt worse. He became more isolated, and although he had previously been a good student, he now found it difficult to concentrate in class. His mind wandered constantly to thoughts of food, and he spent a lot of time planning what he would eat at the next meal.

His friends realized that something was wrong, but no one felt comfortable enough to approach him. On one of his visits home, however, he could no longer hide his eating disorder from his parents. He was pale, thin and appeared to be ill. His mood was depressed. The next morning his parents took him to the family doctor, who made the diagnosis of anorexia nervosa.

Incidence Among Males

The number of men with body image concerns has increased greatly, but the possibility of eating disorders in men is still not receiving the attention it deserves. Doctors now believe that at least 10 percent of individuals with eating disorders are male. It is true that in general most men are not as concerned as women about pursuing thinness, but men are concerned with body shape, size and the development of muscles. In men, cultural ideals relating to muscularity may contribute to low self-esteem and poor body image. Men who participate in bodybuilding are at greater risk for body image or eating problems. Eating disorders such as anorexia and bulimia are more common in men participating in sports requiring a low body weight, such as wrestling and gymnastics. In addition, although eating disorders occur in many heterosexual men, there is a higher incidence of eating disorders amongst homosexual men because of the high value placed on appearance in the male gay community.

As we are learning to look for and recognize the symptoms in males, we have come to realize that the incidence of eating disorders is much higher than we once believed it to be. Just as there is pressure on women to achieve an ideal body image, so is there increasing pressure on men to achieve a cultural ideal. Most of the underlying issues that cause eating disorders are similar for both men and women. Almost all suffer from low self-esteem.

Which Eating Disorders Occur in Males?

ANOREXIA NERVOSA

Anorexia nervosa is not common among males, but it does occur. The diagnosis of anorexia nervosa in males depends on the same criteria as in females, apart from the symptom of loss of menstruation. Males, too, may become dangerously thin, may see themselves as fat even as they continue to lose weight, and may exercise obsessively. In addition, they may sometimes binge, vomit, or misuse laxatives, diuretics or diet pills. Males exposed to sports and activities requiring thinness are at greater risk of developing anorexia nervosa. Examples of these activities are wrestling, athletics, gymnastics and ski-jumping. In both females and males, anorexia is often triggered by dieting, but males usually start dieting for specific reasons, rather than because of a cultural condoning of thinness.

Men will often diet to improve their performance in athletics, to make weight for wrestling or gymnastics, for health reasons, or to try to improve a relationship.

As with women, once anorexia nervosa sets in, several factors keep it going, including initial positive reinforcement because of the weight loss.

BULIMIA NERVOSA

Symptoms of bulimia include recurrent episodes of binge eating, followed by some method of trying to rid the body of the excess calories from the binge. This may involve vomiting, dieting, excessive exercising, or the misuse of laxatives, diuretics, or diet pills. In men as in women, bulimia is more common than anorexia nervosa.

BINGE-EATING DISORDER

Binge-eating disorder, which used to be known as compulsive overeating, is now recognized as an eating disorder, but has not yet been formally classified as one. People with binge-eating disorder engage in regular episodes of bingeing, at which time they eat very large amounts of food in a short period of time, with a feeling of being out of control. Unlike bulimia, binges are not followed by purging, although people with binge-eating disorder may have frequent failed attempts at weight loss. It occurs in about two men for every three women, which is a higher male-to-female ratio than in the other eating disorders. As is the case with other eating disorders, binge-eating disorder is associated with depression and anxiety in both men and women.

EATING DISORDER NOT OTHERWISE SPECIFIED

Many males have eating disorders that may not fit the strict criteria of the specific eating disorders mentioned above, but can still have harmful consequences. Such problems should also be taken seriously and treated appropriately.

Body Image Problems

BODY DYSMORPHIC DISORDER

Body dysmorphic disorder, also known as body dysmorphia, is a condition where there is excessive preoccupation with a very small or imagined defect in physical appearance. It occurs in males as well as females. It seems to run in families, although psychological and sociocultural factors play a role in its cause. Men and women who suffer with this compare themselves to idealistic images of beauty and feel they don't measure up. They may focus obsessively on one aspect of their bodies, for example their face, nose, arms or chests, and may develop repetitive behaviors such as repeated checking in mirrors.

The concern about their appearance occupies much of their time, and can severely affect their day-to-day living. They develop low self-esteem, become more and more self-conscious, and often withdraw from social activity. Some request plastic surgery. The disorder is serious, and patients may become severely depressed and even attempt suicide.

Body dysmorphic disorder often begins in adolescence, although it may develop earlier. Unfortunately, a diagnosis may be delayed by lack of knowledge about the condition, or embarrassment on behalf of the patients. Treatment includes some form of psychotherapy, e.g., cognitive behavioral therapy; education about the illness; and medications when appropriate.

Muscle dysmorphia, also known as reverse anorexia, is probably a type of body dysmorphic disorder. It is a condition that occurs mostly in men. People with muscle dysmorphia believe they are never big and muscular enough. They are preoccupied with their build, which they imagine to be small, though in reality it is often large and muscular. They may abuse anabolic steroids. Muscle dysmorphia has similarities to eating disorders. In anorexia nervosa, the person never feels thin enough; in muscle dysmorphia, he never feels muscular enough.

What Causes Eating Disorders in Men?

The causes in men are similar to the causes in women. (See chapter 3.) A combination of factors often play a role. Those factors may include the following.

GENETICS

Family and twin studies indicate that eating disorders tend to run in families.

PERSONALITY

Individuals with eating disorders tend to have certain distinctive personality traits. They tend to have perfectionistic attitudes, and usually suffer from low self-esteem.

FAMILY

Family problems and stress can be either a contributing factor or a result of the eating disorder, or both. A number of family factors can put an individual at risk. These include depression in a parent, stress such as divorce or loss, a family history of an eating disorder, poor communication and inability to deal with conflict, and perfectionistic attitudes.

STRESSFUL LIFE EVENTS

Sometimes a particularly stressful event, such as leaving home for college, may be the beginning of an eating disorder. Probably more common, however, is a history of stressful events, which may include abuse.

SOCIAL AND CULTURAL ENVIRONMENT

As we discussed, although men are not usually as concerned about becoming thin as are women, they are still exposed to strong cultural messages about being fit and muscular. Our culture and the media endorse increasing muscularity for men, and men, like women, do seem to be sensitive to media messages. They are also bombarded with ads about fitness products, machines to build stronger muscles, and products to lose fat and gain muscle. The men in today's fitness ads are far more muscular than they were years ago. Even children's toy action figures have become more muscular. Although some men wish to lose weight and others prefer to gain weight, most strive for bigger muscles or more well-defined muscles.

Research has shown that men are less happy about their own bodies after looking at what they believe to be attractive male bodies, and were more satisfied with their bodies after looking at less attractive ones. Clearly, some men measure their bodies against cultural ideas. Unfortunately, these ideals are often impossible to achieve, and some men have resorted to using anabolic steroids, which can result in dangerous side effects.

OTHER FACTORS

Other factors that may put males at increased risk include the following:

- A history of being overweight.
- A history of being teased.
- Certain sports, including gymnastics, athletics, wrestling, skiing and body-building. Male runners may be at increased risk for developing anorexia nervosa.
- Depression.
- A history of abuse.
- Gay orientation. Studies have shown that gay men have a higher incidence of body image problems, eating disturbances and eating disorders than heterosexual men. Part of this may be caused by their increased valuation of thinness. Note: Most males with eating disorders do not have a gay orientation.
- Low self-esteem and poor body image.
- Dieting.

Why Do We See Fewer Males with Eating Disorders?

We are unsure whether men are genetically or biologically less prone to eating disorders, or if they are protected because they are less exposed to social pressures promoting thinness. Girls and women are under more pressure to be thin than are boys and men. This difference is probably mostly due to the cultural value placed on female thinness and its association with beauty. Another important difference is that during puberty, which is the time when eating disordered behavior often begins to develop, girls start changing away from their cultural ideal. Their bodies become more curved, and they may develop more body fat. These changes, in a susceptible person, can contribute to a poor body image and dieting. Boys, on the other hand, approach their "ideal" as they become more muscular after puberty. On the other hand, although males in our society have not been as concerned about thinness, many are concerned about body shape and muscularity. Some want to increase their weight, and some want to lose weight.

Though eating disorders occur less often in men, many cases of eating disorders in men also go untreated for the following reasons:

• Men may not go for treatment because they fear the stigma attached to males with eating disorders.

• Unlike women with anorexia nervosa who develop amenorrhea, men don't develop any specific signal that something is wrong, so the diagnosis may be delayed.

• Because anorexia nervosa is less common in men, clinicians may not make the diagnosis initially.

• Many programs don't accept males into treatment.

Signs That a Male May Have an Eating Disorder

Some of these signs can be caused by other problems, so it is always best to get checked by a doctor to confirm the diagnosis of an eating disorder.

• Weight loss or gain, not explained by another illness
• Weight fluctuating significantly
• Continuing to diet in spite of being a normal or low weight
• Excessive concern about your weight or shape
• Being preoccupied about food, calories and weight
• Feeling fat when others say you are thin
• Recurrent episodes of binge eating (eating very large amounts of food in a short period of time in an out-of-control manner)
• Shame and embarrassment about the amount of food eaten
• Vomiting after eating in order to prevent weight gain
• Using laxatives, diuretics or diet pills to prevent weight gain
• Feeling that your self-worth is tied in to the way you look
• Low self-esteem
• Difficulty in thinking or concentrating
• Depressed mood

Complications

Complications of eating disorders in men are similar to those in women. Eating disorders can affect almost every organ system in the body. Some of the complications that may occur in males are listed below.

MEDICAL COMPLICATIONS

- Malnutrition.
- Heart problems.
- Electrolyte abnormalities.
- Muscle weakness and wasting.
- Gastrointestinal problems.
- Dental caries (cavities).
- Kidney abnormalities.
- Brain changes.
- Osteoporosis. We have come to learn that males with eating disorders such as anorexia nervosa are also at risk for developing thinning of the bones and osteoporosis.
- Delayed sexual development.
- Decreased levels of testosterone.

PSYCHOLOGICAL COMPLICATIONS

- Poor body image and low self-esteem.
- Poor concentration.
- Social isolation.
- Negative effects on all aspects of life, including work, social life, and relationships.

There may also be associated psychiatric problems, such as depression, anxiety disorders, substance abuse or obsessive-compulsive disorder. Often obsessive-compulsive, anxiety or depressive symptoms will improve once the eating disorder is treated. (See chapter 8 for more detail.)

Treatment

Treatment of eating disorders in men, as is the case in women, involves:

- Medical care
- Nutritional rehabilitation
- Psychotherapy—individual, family or group
- Medication, when appropriate

Men often start dieting at a lower body fat percentage than do women, so they may develop the complications of starvation earlier on in the illness. As is the case in women, the first goal of therapy is to restore normal weight and to treat complications. Once normal weight has been restored, therapy focuses on issues such as regulating eating behavior, improving body image and self-esteem, diminishing anxiety, improving coping skills, and improving relationships. (See chapter 9 for details.) As patients get better it can often be helpful to begin resistance exercises gradually. This helps men and women feel better about their bodies as they regain weight, and can also help tremendously with morale.

Men are at risk for all the serious complications of eating disorders we see in women. It is not unusual for patients with anorexia nervosa to need hospitalization at some time during their illness. One big problem is the lack of facilities that accept men into treatment. Another problem is the lack of expertise and sensitivity in dealing with male patients. Researchers hope that increasing awareness will solve these problems.

Specific treatments for some eating disorders are listed below.

ANOREXIA NERVOSA

Treatment usually consists of nutritional rehabilitation, education, and individual, group or family counseling. Medications may be used to treat associated problems such as anxiety or depression, but should usually only be started once weight has been restored. Men with anorexia nervosa may require more calories because they normally have more lean body mass than women do. They may also need to gain larger amounts of weight to get back to normal weight.

Bulimia Nervosa

The initial goal of treatment is to have the individual eat regular healthy meals, maintain a healthy weight and stop purging. Treatment includes nutritional counseling and some form of therapy. Cognitive behavioral therapy, which focuses on understanding behaviors and learning new behaviors, is very effective for people suffering with bulimia. Medications such as Prozac may be used to treat associated problems such as depression or anxiety, or to reduce the urge to binge.

Binge-Eating Disorder

As in the case of bulimia, the goal is to regulate eating, prevent bingeing, and maintain a healthy weight. Another important part of treatment is to work on self-esteem issues and relationship issues. Treatment usually involves psychotherapy and education about the illness. Medications are used when appropriate.

A Message for Young Males

Your body's size and shape has nothing to do with who you are as a person. Focus on your good qualities and take pride in achievements other than those related to appearance. Spend time with friends who accept and appreciate you for who you really are, not for the way you look. Those are your true friends.

An eating disorder is not a "female illness." Eating disorders are being recognized more and more frequently in males today.

Get professional help if you:

- Spend a great deal of time worrying about your weight or shape
- Are dieting in spite of being thin
- Skip meals
- Purge or use medications to lose weight
- Regularly eat in an out-of-control way
- Exercise excessively

- Have low self-esteem
- Have a depressed mood

Eating disorders are treatable, and the earlier you get appropriate treatment, the better the outcome.

6

Warning Signs of an Eating Disorder

Eating disorders can result in serious medical and psychological complications. The 'eath rate of young women with anorexia nervosa is twelve times that of young women without the illness. Because eating disorders are so prevalent in America, and because they know no age, sex, class or race boundaries, it is important to recognize some of their early warning signs. The earlier an eating disorder is diagnosed and treated appropriately, the better the outcome for the patient.

Unfortunately, in many instances, eating disorders go undiagnosed for long periods of time. While it is often difficult to hide anorexia nervosa because of the obvious weight loss, people with bulimia may be of normal weight without any obvious signs of illness. In addition, sufferers of bulimia feel tremendous shame related to their bingeing and purging, and in spite of the fact that binge eating and purging behaviors are common in young people, each sufferer feels very alone. Young people with bulimia nervosa may struggle with the disorder for months or even years before seeking professional help. Very often even parents are unaware of the problem until late into the illness.

The Ross Daughters' Story

Mr. and Mrs. Ross have two teenage daughters, and Mr. Ross, who learned of my interest in eating disorders, recently told me his story. Amy, the oldest daughter, appeared to be good at everything she set her mind on doing, and that included schoolwork, debating, sports and music. Her sister Michelle was a good student and good all-rounder too, but was regularly compared to Amy when she didn't quite make the grade. She also didn't consider herself as pretty as her sister was. No one else was really aware of her feelings.

Their parents cared deeply about both their daughters. Although Michelle seemed quieter and spent more time alone, they didn't notice any particular problem. Both daughters went to an out-of-state college, and six months after Michelle began college, Mr. Ross received a call from the headmaster, who said that he suspected that Michelle had an eating disorder. Michelle was brought home, ten pounds thinner than when she had left home, and was taken to a physician for assessment. She later admitted to having engaged in binge eating and vomiting for two years. No one had had a clue about this.

How Do You Know If Someone Close to You Has an Eating Disorder?

Many parents, caretakers and teachers ask me this question, and others sadly tell me that they missed the early signs in their own children until it was too late. It is sometimes extremely difficult for anyone to pick up the early warning signs. Teenagers may go to great lengths to hide their illness. We have already discussed the secretiveness of patients with bulimia. Patients with anorexia nervosa may try to disguise their weight loss by wearing baggy clothes or hiding weights or large numbers of coins in their clothes when being weighed. They may hide their dieting behavior by not sitting with the family at mealtimes or by busying themselves with the preparation of food, without eating any of the meal themselves.

The following are some clues that may indicate that a person has anorexia nervosa, bulimia nervosa or binge-eating disorder.

ANOREXIA NERVOSA

- Unexplained weight loss, or not gaining weight as expected
- Feeling fat in spite of being thin
- Continued dieting in spite of excessive weight loss
- Denial of hunger
- Development of food rituals such as cutting up food a certain way
- In women, loss of menstrual periods
- Excessive preoccupation with dieting, weight and shape
- Feeling cold when others do not
- Hair loss
- Layer of fine downy hair covering face and body (lanugo)
- Excessive exercising
- Low self-esteem
- Social withdrawal
- Weakness
- Difficulty concentrating

BULIMIA NERVOSA

- Regular episodes of binge eating: eating large amounts of food in a short period of time
- Feeling out of control during episodes of bingeing
- Mysterious disappearance of large amounts of food
- Telltale signs of a binge such as wrappers or empty food containers
- Dieting between episodes of "binge eating"
- Preoccupation with body weight and shape
- Complaints of being fat
- Evidence of vomiting after meals
- Evidence of using non-prescribed laxatives or diuretics
- Weight fluctuations
- Secretive behavior
- Heartburn in a young person
- Frequent and extended bathroom use after eating
- Swollen or tender parotid glands
- Dental caries or loss of dental enamel
- Calluses on hands and knuckles from inducing vomiting

- Constant complaints of sore throat
- Social withdrawal
- Low self-esteem

Note that a person with bulimia may be of low weight, normal weight or even slightly overweight.

Binge-Eating Disorder

- Regular attempts at dieting
- Skipping meals
- Regular episodes of eating large amounts of food in a short period of time
- Feeling out of control during episodes of eating
- Using food to cope with daily problems and stress
- Hiding food for binges
- Frequently feeling full or bloated
- Constipation
- Feeling guilty about eating
- Low self-esteem
- Social withdrawal or isolation
- Depressed mood

A person with binge-eating disorder is often overweight.

Could You Have an Eating Disorder?

There is often overlap of symptoms between the different eating disorders. Not all symptoms fit neatly into one diagnosis every time. Sometimes, someone with anorexia nervosa may go on to develop bulimia, and vice versa.

You may have an eating disorder if you:

- have low self-esteem
- constantly worry about your weight
- weigh yourself frequently

- diet or skip meals
- see yourself as fat even when people say you are thin
- regularly eat large amounts of food with the feeling of being out of control
- feel guilty about eating
- believe that the way you look is related to your value as a person
- exercise excessively
- vomit or use laxatives, diuretics, or diet pills after eating to try to lose weight

It is important to know that some of the above symptoms found in people with anorexia, bulimia or binge-eating disorder may occur in conditions other than eating disorders. Someone with weight loss may have depression; weight loss and irregular periods may signal thyroid disease; a person with heartburn and vomiting could have reflux. It is up to a good physician to make a correct diagnosis.

One key difference in someone who has an eating disorder is that he or she is not satisfied with a healthy weight, and has a fear of gaining weight, whereas the person without an eating disorder is usually satisfied with reaching a healthy weight goal. The self-image of someone with an eating disorder is closely tied in to his or her personal appearance, and that person will also have an unhealthy relationship with food.

If you have an eating disorder, or wonder whether you may have an eating disorder, I urge you to get help as soon as possible. Symptoms often get worse if not treated, and you can't fix this by yourself. Part of the process of getting help will be learning more about eating disorders and how they may affect you. You will learn more about nutrition and about yourself.

What about a friend or family member? What should you do if you suspect that a friend or someone close to you might have an eating disorder? Here are some do's and don'ts.

Do approach the person in private.

Do be supportive and caring.

Do tell the person that you are available to listen and to try to help.

Do encourage the person to seek professional help. You don't have control over whether they go for help, but by being there, listening, and offering your support, you can make a difference, and perhaps give them the incentive to take the next step to getting well.

Do speak to a counselor, doctor, teacher or another trusted adult if you are still concerned.

Don't be critical.
Don't be judgmental.
Don't try to fix this by yourself. The person needs professional help.

How a Friend Helped

Theresa, an eighteen-year-old premedical student, noticed a big change in her friend Sonya. Her weight was fluctuating up and down, and she frequently made excuses in order to skip meals. One night Theresa found evidence that her friend had vomited after dinner. Although Sonya continued attending all her classes, she slowly withdrew from her friends and most social functions. Theresa was very worried about the possibility that Sonya might have bulimia, and she approached Sonya one day with an offer to help. She was not quite ready for the harsh response. Sonya told her that there was no problem and that she did not need help. In spite of the brush-off, Theresa left a piece of paper with the name and number of a center specializing in eating disorders. She didn't have much hope that Sonya would ever look at the paper.

Sonya didn't—for a while. However, her eating disorder worsened. A few months later, she was bingeing and vomiting daily. She found herself more and more isolated, and although she had been a conscientious student in the past, she now frequently missed classes. Her relationships were suffering, as her time was spent obsessing about food and planning meals and binges. She was exhausted and depressed and felt that no one would understand. That's when she picked up the piece of paper that Theresa had left her and made that first call. She told me: "That was the most difficult thing to do—that phone call. I wasn't ready to accept help before, but I think Theresa saved my life."

Understanding more about eating disorders and learning of their warning signs can help you recognize symptoms in others and perhaps in yourself. Hopefully this will lead to an earlier diagnosis, earlier treatment and a better outcome.

7

Complications of Eating Disorders

Eating disorders must be taken seriously. They are serious illnesses that can affect almost every organ system in the body. Anorexia nervosa, in fact, has the highest premature death rate of any psychiatric disorder. Every person suffering with an eating disorder is affected in some way both physically and psychologically, though some people may seem to remain relatively stable, while others suffer more severe consequences.

The sooner someone comes for treatment, the better, and the sooner they can receive education about their disorder and its serious complications (many of which we are still learning about) the better chance we have of having a good outcome. Young girls and boys who are dieting excessively may not be aware of the long-term effects of malnutrition, some of which may not be reversible. This chapter will discuss some of the complications of eating disorders.

Personal Stories

KERRY'S STORY

Kerry was one of the "popular" girls in middle school. She seemed to have it all—a loving family, good grades and good looks. Kerry didn't always feel that way about herself, though. She worked very hard to get her A's, and she was always afraid of disappointing her parents, who were both high achievers. Kerry also didn't feel that her looks measured up to those of many of her friends. She would have liked to be thinner and more athletic.

Then something happened that devastated Kerry and shocked the neighborhood and family friends. Her parents, most unexpectedly, decided to separate. Kerry felt that her world was shattered and that she had very little control over her life. Her dad moved out, and she and her mother were alone. She started finding comfort in eating. Late at night when her mom was asleep, she would go down into the kitchen and eat whatever she could find. She felt sick and ashamed afterwards, but found comfort in sleep. This scenario repeated itself night after night, with Kerry eating very little during the day. One night, when she felt especially full after eating, she vomited, and was surprised to feel some relief. This began the dangerous cycle of bingeing, then vomiting, and restricting food by day.

Within three months Kerry was vomiting several times a day, and in spite of trying to cover up with cleaning and perfume, she was still leaving telltale signs all over. When her mother realized what was going on, she immediately took Kerry to her primary care physician. Lab tests confirmed that Kerry's electrolyte levels were dangerously abnormal from vomiting, and she was admitted to hospital for rehydration and further treatment.

SARAH'S STORY

Sarah was a fifteen-year-old young woman, who was struggling with a combination of anorexia nervosa and bulimia. In spite of having read about the more serious complications and long term effects of eating disorders, she was most worried that her cheeks were getting "fatter." This occurs as a result of the salivary gland enlargement that is seen with bingeing and vomiting. She was less concerned about heart complications, gastrointestinal complications or the very common side effect of osteoporosis, as she did not think these could happen to someone like her. Sarah had had the disorder for a number of years. It was especially sad because she seemed to have very little motivation to get well. I heard later that she spoke to two plastic surgeons about having her cheeks made "thinner." Luckily, they both talked her out of the procedure, and she was encouraged instead to continue therapy for her eating disorder.

STACY'S STORY

Stacy was a sixteen-year-old girl with anorexia nervosa who had to be hospitalized after she lost weight very rapidly and became dehydrated. She developed abdominal pain while in hospital and was found to have gallstones, which are sometimes a result of excessive weight loss and dehydration. Luckily she was operated on without problems. She continued with therapy after she was dismissed from the hospital, and she has done very well.

All of these stories are true, and they show only a few of the many possible problems that eating disorders can produce. Let's look at some others.

Malnutrition

The human body requires a certain number of calories and a certain amount of fat to maintain normal metabolic and endocrine functions and allow for growth and repair. A certain number of calories is also required for someone to maintain a normal healthy weight. What is a healthy weight? The number of pounds varies from person to person, but a normal, healthy weight is one at which all systems of the body are functioning normally. At a health weight a person is able to function well and be free from food obsessions.

Without enough calories and fat, metabolic processes begin to shut down in order to save energy. Without food, the body breaks down its own muscle tissue to use as fuel. The heart rate slows down, blood pressure drops, circulation becomes poor, menstruation may cease, and muscles, including the heart muscle, become weaker. Medications cannot treat the underlying problem. The first step of treatment is providing adequate calories and restoring weight to a healthy level.

Endocrine and Hormonal Problems

A common problem associated with eating disorders is irregular or absent menstruation. When women lose a significant amount of weight, estrogen is decreased, and their menstrual periods become irregular or stop altogether. This can put them at increased risk for developing thinning of the bones (osteoporosis). Menstrual periods usually return in most women with anorexia nervosa when they regain weight to within 90 percent of their ideal body weight, but periods may be delayed in some women in spite of reaching normal weight.

Males may have decreased testosterone. Both boys and girls may have delayed puberty.

Thyroid hormone levels may be low. This is related to starvation.

Osteoporosis

If you have an eating disorder, you are at increased risk of developing osteoporosis or thinning of the bones. Low bone mass, as found in osteoporosis, leads to fragile bones and an increased risk of developing fractures. This happens more often with anorexia nervosa, but it can also occur in the case of bulimia, especially in people with a history of being underweight. Both males and females can be affected. In anorexia nervosa, the bones that are usually affected are the lumbar spine and the hip.

Most of our skeletal bone growth occurs during childhood and the teenage years. Unfortunately, it is during these years that eating disorders often begin.

The following can contribute to or aggravate osteoporosis in people with anorexia nervosa:

- Low weight
- Decreased body fat
- Low intake of of calcium and Vitamin D
- High cortisol levels
- Low levels of estrogen (or testosterone)

Besides eating disorders, the following problems can also put a person at risk for osteoporosis:

- An inadequate diet
- Smoking
- A low level of physical activity and weight-bearing exercise
- Long duration of amenorrhea (lack of menstruation)

With advances in our ability to measure bone density we know that osteoporosis is very common among patients with anorexia nervosa, more so than in those with bulimia. This is a serious condition, and the most effective way to prevent further decline in bone mass is to restore the patient's weight. However, prevention is still far better than cure, as even with treatment, bone mass may only increase by 1 to 5 percent.

Osteoporosis in someone with an eating disorder is treated by restoring nutrition and weight and prescribing weight-bearing exercises and supplemental calcium and vitamin D as needed. Low estrogen levels may contribute to the bone loss, but replacing estrogen has not (to date) been shown to prevent or correct the problem in young people with eating disorders. After many years of maintaining a normal weight, osteoporosis may improve.

Now that we are more aware about osteoporosis, we can look for it in people at risk and begin treatment earlier.

What's the best way to prevent osteoporosis? Maintain a normal healthy weight; get enough calcium in your diet; and make sure you get a moderate amount of safe exercise, including weight-bearing exercise. Weight-bearing exercise is anything where your body must bear its own weight, such as walking or aerobic dance. (Swimming is not a weight-bearing exercise because the water bears your weight for you.)

Growth Delay or Short Stature

Young people who do not get adequate nutrition may have stunted bone development and growth delay. If anorexia nervosa begins before or during a young person's growth spurt, that person may lose height. Teenagers with anorexia nervosa can be up to an inch shorter than what they would have been if they had maintained a normal weight.

Electrolyte Abnormalities

Repeated vomiting or the use of laxatives or diuretics may lead to dehydration and electrolyte problems such as low potassium, for example. This can result in serious disturbances in heart rhythm. Dehydration and electrolyte disturbances can also be associated with kidney problems, including kidney failure. Electrolyte abnormalities may cause symptoms such as weakness, constipation, dizziness or leg cramps.

Heart Problems

The singer Karen Carpenter died of cardiac problems caused by her eating disorder in the 1980s. Unfortunately, heart problems are not unusual among patients with eating disorders, and are the cause of death particularly in patients with anorexia nervosa, but also in patients with bulimia. With starvation, heart muscle, like other muscles, is broken down to provide fuel for the body. Heart rate slows down, and blood pressure drops. This can lead to dizziness or fainting. Some people have asked me whether having such a slow heart rate could be a good thing. After all, they say, Olympic athletes have really slow heart rates. In the case of someone with anorexia nervosa, however, the heart rate is low because the heart has become smaller and weaker. Athletes, in contrast, have strong, muscular, efficient hearts. Patients with eating disorders may develop heart failure or heart rhythm disturbances from electrolyte abnormalities. Exercise in extremely underweight patients is dangerous, because if the heart is not functioning properly, it can't supply the tissues with adequate oxygen during exercise.

What increases a person's risk for heart problems?

- Severe rapid weight loss
- Frequent purging
- Abuse of ipecac to cause vomiting
- Having another illness such as diabetes
- Being older

Gastrointestinal Problems

Patients with bulimia nervosa may have swelling of the salivary glands. They may also complain of sore throat, difficulty swallowing, hoarseness or heartburn, as repeated vomiting causes irritation of the esophagus from stomach acids. An esophageal tear may also occur. A symptom of esophageal tears is vomiting of blood.

With anorexia nervosa, stomach function becomes impaired with malnutrition. Stomach emptying is delayed, which means that food leaves the stomach more slowly. This causes the individual to feel full or bloated after even small meals. It can also cause nausea, reflux and vomiting. People with anorexia may have constipation, which can be due to inadequate calorie intake, and can be aggravated by laxative abuse. These symptoms improve as patients are nourished and become well. Unless constipation becomes severe, it is usually treated with only fluids and added fiber in the diet.

Metabolic Problems

With starvation, the body slows down to conserve energy. Circulation is slowed. Low heart rate, low blood pressure, dizziness and even fainting may occur. In some people heart rates are as low as 30 to 40. Patients with anorexia have a low body temperature and may therefore feel cold all the time. Many patients with anorexia nervosa may notice a bluish-purple discoloration of their hands and feet. Blood glucose may be very low because of starvation.

Damage to Muscles

As muscle is broken down for fuel, muscle weakness and muscle wasting occurs. The heart, which is also a muscle, becomes smaller and weaker.

High Cholesterol

This may come as a surprise to you, but cholesterol levels are usually high in anorexia.

Dental Caries (Cavities)

Tooth enamel may be eroded from exposure to acid caused by vomiting. People with bulimia frequently develop dental caries and should be followed by a dentist regularly.

Damage to Bone Marrow

Even the bone marrow may be affected with starvation. This results in decreased red blood cells (important for carrying oxygen); white blood cells (important for fighting infection, although we do not know if a low white cell count increases the risk of infection); and platelets (important for helping blood clotting and preventing bleeding).

Brain Changes

Both thinking and concentration are impaired with starvation. Patients with anorexia nervosa may have changes in the brain, which have been demonstrated by new brain scanning techniques. Most of these abnormalities seem to reverse as patients gain weight. We are still unsure whether any of the changes are permanent.

Infertility

There appears to be an increased incidence of infertility and obstetric complications in people with eating disorders, especially anorexia nervosa. However, some patients with anorexia nervosa do become pregnant and do deliver healthy babies. If a woman with an eating disorder becomes pregnant, it is important for her to be followed regularly, not only by her obstetrician, but also by an eating disorder specialist.

Damage to Skin and Hair

With starvation, patients can develop thinning of the hair and drying of the nails. Many notice a fine, thin layer of hair on their faces or bodies, known as "lanugo hair." Calluses or abrasions may develop on hands and fingers from the trauma from teeth when fingers are used to cause vomiting.

Damage to Eyes

Patients sometimes develop burst blood vessels in or around the eye from the increased pressure from vomiting. Rarely, retinal detachment can occur.

In summary, every organ system of the body can be affected by starvation, including the liver, the kidneys and the endocrine system.

Physical Complications Associated with Specific Eating Disorders

The following are some of the medical complications of each specific eating disorder:

ANOREXIA NERVOSA

- The heart becomes smaller and weaker. Heart rate and blood pressure drop. There is an increased risk of developing heart rhythm disturbances and heart failure.
- Absent menstruation.
- Osteoporosis.
- Dehydration, which can lead to kidney problems and kidney failure.
- Muscle weakness.
- Delayed emptying of the stomach and constipation.
- Dry skin.
- Dry hair and hair loss.
- Weakness.
- Other problems, including decreased immunity, obstetric problems, thyroid problems.

BULIMIA NERVOSA

- Electrolyte abnormalities (from purging) that can lead to heart rhythm disturbances and even heart failure.
- Reflux.
- Gastrointestinal problems, including diarrhea or constipation.
- Tears or rupture of the esophagus from repeated vomiting.
- Dental problems from repeated exposure of the teeth to stomach acids during vomiting.

BINGE-EATING DISORDER

Patients with binge-eating disorder who are overweight may have complications related to obesity. These include:

- High blood pressure.
- Elevated cholesterol levels.
- Heart problems.
- Joint problems.
- Diabetes.

LAXATIVE ABUSE

Unfortunately, a number of individuals with bulimia abuse laxatives. Their rationale is that with laxatives you can prevent weight gain by causing diarrhea and preventing food from being absorbed. The truth is that laxatives do not play much of a role in preventing weight gain. What looks like weight loss is mostly water loss, as laxatives work lower down in the bowel, after most of the food has already been absorbed. Also, laxative abuse can be very dangerous. Abuse can result in dehydration, electrolyte abnormalities and bleeding, amongst other problems.

Psychological and Psychiatric Problems

Patients with eating disorders are plagued with thoughts about food and weight. This preoccupation eventually begins to affect their physical and mental well-being. They almost always have low self-esteem, and in the case of bulimia and binge-eating disorder, they experience shame about their eating behaviors. Many people with anorexia nervosa develop obsessions, compulsions, and rituals, many of which go away as their weight approaches normal. Depression and anxiety are often associated with an eating disorder, and suicide is a serious risk. Unfortunately, some patients become addicted to drugs and alcohol, which makes treatment more complicated.

SUZANNE'S STORY

Suzanne told me she spent every morning at school in fear, dreading the thought of having to eat lunch in front of her friends. It was hard for her to concentrate in class while thoughts about what she would eat and where she would eat were constantly on her mind. Many days she chose not to eat lunch at all, and other days she hid behind one of the bookshelves to eat her sandwich. It took a month before a friend expressed concern about her and somehow convinced her to go for help. Today, years later, Suzanne tries to help other young people in similar situations.

EFFECT ON RELATIONSHIPS

People with eating disorders often become socially withdrawn or even isolated. The preoccupation with food, calories and weight takes up an enormous part of their lives and drains their energy. One young girl told me that she had almost no time left to do anything else. Dealing with three meals a day, worrying between meals, preparing food, and weighing herself took up all her time. She certainly had no time for a boyfriend. Relationships with friends suffer. Someone with an eating disorder may feel that she has nothing in common with her friends or that they may not understand.

People struggling with eating disorders can also be overwhelmed by social gatherings of large groups of people, especially when eating is involved. Often they will avoid these functions.

Eating disorders affect family relationships. There is so much focus placed on the illness. It increases tension and can cause conflict in the family. It strains family relationships. Parents and siblings may feel scared, angry and confused.

In summary, the complications of eating disorders can seem overwhelming. I did not include this chapter to scare you. I think it is important for young people to be aware of the physical and mental consequences of eating disorders. It is also reasonable for you to be very hopeful, because in spite of the complications of eating disorders, good treatment is available, and young people seem to do especially well.

8

Associated Disorders

A variety of psychological or psychiatric disorders may coexist in people with eating disorders. In some people these problems may have been present before the eating disorder began, while in others they may be associated with the eating disorder. In many people, once the eating disorder is under control, some symptoms of the other disorders improve. Other symptoms may require further treatment.

The following are some of the problems that may be associated with eating disorders:

- Mood disorders
- Anxiety disorders
- Obsessive compulsive disorder
- Substance abuse
- Personality disorders
- Posttraumatic stress disorder
- Self-injury

Mood Disorders and Depression

We find an increased incidence of major depression and other mood disorders among people with eating disorders. There is a clear association between eating disorders and depression. People who are underweight or have binge eating and vomiting may suffer from depression, and on the other hand people with depression may either overeat or lose weight. Also, a significant number of people with eating disorders have a family history of depression.

Because malnutrition and weight loss may cause symptoms of depression, it is sometimes difficult to know if there is underlying depression or if the depression has occurred because of the eating disorder. If the latter is the case, symptoms will improve as the eating disorder is brought under control.

Rhona's Story

Rhona, a fifteen-year-old young woman, was seen at an eating disorder center because of weight loss and a depressed mood. She was diagnosed as having anorexia nervosa and was begun on individual and family therapy. As her weight approached normal, her depression resolved without medication.

Susan's Story

On the other hand, fourteen-year-old Susan, who had an eating disorder with weight loss and depression, continued to have symptoms of depression when she regained weight. She was successfully treated with antidepressants.

Symptoms of depression may include the following (symptoms are usually persistent over a period of time):

- Feelings of sadness, hopelessness or worthlessness.
- Irritability.
- Agitation.
- Lack of energy.
- Loss of interest in activities once enjoyed.
- Change in sleep or eating pattern.
- Change in weight—either loss or gain.
- Difficulty with concentration.
- Social withdrawal.
- Poor school performance.

- Suicidal thoughts.
- Abuse of drugs or alcohol.

How does one tell the difference between someone who is sad and someone who is depressed? After all, everyone experiences a sad mood from time to time. You might be sad, for example, when you have to say goodbye to someone you love, when a pet dies, when you do poorly in a test, or when someone has disappointed you. The difference is that a sad mood is temporary, whereas depression usually persists, requires treatment, and if severe, can seriously affect one's quality of living.

Depression is a serious illness that should be taken seriously. It usually won't just go away by itself. If you believe you are depressed, it is important to get professional help as soon as possible. If you have suicidal thoughts, call 911 or go to the nearest emergency room. Remember that however hopeless you may feel, help is available. Depression can be treated successfully.

Anxiety Disorders

The prevalence of anxiety disorders in general seems to be higher for people with anorexia nervosa and bulimia nervosa than for the general population. Anxiety disorders are serious medical conditions that significantly interfere with quality of life. This is not the same as the anxiety we all feel before an exam or a first date. It is a chronic anxiety that often persists or gets worse without treatment.

Symptoms may include:

- Persistent anxiety or worry.
- Irritability.
- Restlessness.
- Sleep disturbances.
- Panic attacks.

Panic Disorder (Panic Attacks)

A panic attack can be terrifying, and is associated with intense fear or anxiety, sweating, a racing pulse, a feeling of being short of breath, and chest pain. Panic attacks strike suddenly, without any clear reason and in a variety of situations. Some people experience them while driving on the highway or while taking an exam. Others may experience them at rest in their own homes. They can cause people to develop a fear and an avoidance of certain situations in which the panic attacks might occur. Some people's lives become severely affected and restricted because of the attacks and the fear that they may return. The good news is that many individuals have only one attack that never recurs. Panic attacks affect women more than men, and usually begin in older teenagers or young adults.

If you do suffer from panic disorder, it is important to get professional help. Panic attacks can be treated with medication, cognitive-behavioral therapy and education about panic symptoms. Once again, this is a treatable illness.

Obsessive-Compulsive Disorder

Obsessive compulsive disorder may exist together with anorexia nervosa or bulimia nervosa. Also, many patients with eating disorders may have some obsessive-compulsive symptoms without having a full-blown obsessive-compulsive disorder. Obsessions are persistent thoughts that are unpleasant and inappropriate. Compulsions are repetitive behaviors that are performed to try to reduce distress or prevent an imagined bad event from occurring.

Before she went to bed each night, Mary had to check all the doors in the house six times to be sure that they were locked. She became more and more anxious until she performed the ritual of checking.

Some people check stoves or ovens over and over again. Debby was such a person. She had great difficulty leaving her house. Her compulsive checking of the stove took so much time that she was always late for meetings and other events. Although she knew her obsession was irrational, it would not go away.

A nurse working in a large clinic was obsessed with germs and the fear of being contaminated. She washed her hands for about an hour each morning, and on several occasions came to work late because of the hand-washing. Her hands were raw from scrubbing, and her work began to suffer. It was only after someone discovered that she had stolen tranquilizers to try to self-medicate that she was referred for treatment. After a few months of treatment, her illness is now under control.

Some of these obsessive, obtrusive thoughts go along with an eating disorder, and they may resolve once the person has recovered from the eating disorder. A person with anorexia nervosa may appear to be obsessive. One young girl with anorexia was "obsessed" by the belief that she was going to become fat if she did not exercise for two hours every day. This compelled her to exercise every single day, often to her detriment. Nothing—not homework, social activities or even illness—could keep her from exercising.

If you recognize some of these symptoms in yourself, you don't necessarily have to be concerned. Many healthy people may perform little rituals such as checking the stove or front door a few times before they leave the home. The difference is that for people with obsessive-compulsive disorder, these worries and rituals take up significant time, cause them a lot of distress, and interfere with their lives.

Obsessive-compulsive disorder is treated with medications, cognitive behavioral therapy, or both.

Substance Abuse

Unfortunately, substance abuse or dependence is not unusual in men and women with eating disorders. It is more common among patients with bulimia nervosa than anorexia nervosa, and is usually seen in those who have more problems with impulsivity in general. Initial treatment of the eating disorder and substance abuse is usually done in an eating disorder center which has the capabilities to treat both eating disorders and addiction. Often the addiction is related to the eating disorder and the addiction may lessen when the eating disorder is treated. If this does not happen, referral to an inpatient or outpatient drug rehabilitation center may be necessary.

Personality Disorders

Individuals with anorexia nervosa often have distinctive personality traits, which include being sensitive, self-critical, narcissistic or perfectionistic, or they may have unstable moods, behavior and relationships. Those with bulimia are more likely to be impulsive, have "up and down" moods, or have intense unstable relationships. People who have unstable moods, behaviors and relationships may be more likely to be hospitalized, and often have a poorer outcome.

Posttraumatic Stress Disorder

There seems to be a higher rate of posttraumatic stress disorder among women with bulimia. There is also a higher rate of past sexual abuse, including incest and rape, in teenagers who have bulimia compared to the general population. Most patients with bulimia, however, have no history of sexual abuse.

Self-Injury

Self-injury or self-mutilation is when people intentionally harm themselves without always intending to commit suicide. This serious problem may go hand-in-hand with an eating disorder.

Lori's Story

Lori began cutting her arms and legs with razor blades about six months into her eating disorder. She had a younger sister with a chronic illness, and her parents were recently separated. She was going through tremendous emotional pain in her life. For a long time she hid her terrible secret from her family. It was only when her mother found a used razor blade in Lori's trashcan that she became suspicious. Luckily Lori was taken to her physician for an assessment and treatment, and has learned healthier ways to cope with her pain.

It's hard to understand why people would intentionally inflict pain on themselves. Some people say it relieves their stress. Others say they find it easier to bear physical pain rather than the emotional pain they suffer. One patient stated that she preferred to feel "something" rather than "numbness."

Self-injury is a dangerous and serious problem. If you have this problem, it is important that you get professional help right away.

Treatment for Associated Disorders

When treating people with eating disorders and associated conditions, the eating disorder is generally treated first and weight is restored, as long as the other disorders are not too severe. There are several reasons for treating the eating disorder first. For one thing, after the eating disorder is treated, many of the other symptoms, such as depression, anxiety and obsessions will improve. If the associated condition is treated first, no one will know whether the condition was caused or aggravated by the eating disorder—something that is important to know for proper treatment. Sometimes antidepressants may be used unnecessarily because depression may improve with weight gain alone; and patients may not respond to antidepressant medications when they are starved.

Medical Conditions That Can Complicate Eating Disorders

TYPE 1 DIABETES MELLITUS

People with chronic illnesses such as diabetes seem to be more at risk for developing an eating disorder. Also, someone with diabetes and an eating disorder is at risk for more diabetic-related complications.

Unfortunately, some diabetic patients engage in the dangerous practice of under-dosing their insulin in order to lose weight. If the diabetes is out of control, the person may need to be hospitalized until stable.

PREGNANCY

Although someone with an active eating disorder who is under-weight is less likely to become pregnant, pregnancies do occur. Pregnant women who have eating disorders are at increased risk for complications of pregnancy. Poor nutritional intake, vomiting, or the use of laxatives, diuretics or other pills can all cause complications in the mother or the fetus. Treatment of a pregnant patient with an eating disorder is complicated and requires a team approach. Whenever possible, it is always better for the eating disorder to be treated before a pregnancy. In some women, eating disorder symptoms may seem to resolve during a pregnancy, and then return after delivery.

So, in summary, there are a number of serious conditions that can go along with an eating disorder. It is important that these associated disorders are also recognized and treated appropriately.

9

Treatment

Eating disorders are serious illnesses, but they can be treated!

The earlier a diagnosis is made and appropriate treatment is begun, the better the outcome is likely to be. The treatment of eating disorders requires a comprehensive approach, which includes medical care, nutritional intervention and counseling, psychotherapy, and medication, if needed.

Treatment involves:

• Restoring weight to a healthy level.
• Treating complications and associated medical and psychiatric problems.
• Stopping dangerous behaviors such as bingeing and vomiting.
• Treating psychological symptoms such as low self-esteem, distorted body image and preoccupation with food and weight.
• Teaching better coping skills.
• Preventing relapse.
• Education.
• Extensive monitoring and follow-up.

Why Is Treatment Difficult?

Although a number of treatment strategies are available to someone suffering from an eating disorder, treatment is not easy. One reason is that many patients, especially those with anorexia nervosa, resist treatment, are terrified of gaining weight, losing their coping mechanism and sometimes losing their identity. Also, it is difficult treating teenagers without involvement of the whole family, and often there are difficult family dynamics. Not all family members may be willing to take part in therapy or to change.

Insurance companies have been reluctant to cover costs for the treatment of eating disorders, which are viewed as behavioral disorders. Hopefully this will change in the near future.

Another concern, and something that potentially undermines treatment, is the emergence of "pro-anorexia" websites. These sites actually advocate eating disorders. They instruct viewers, who are often very young people, how to lose more weight, how to throw up, and so on. In spite of having been aware of these sites, I was horrified when I visited one. There is much debate among psychologists about whether these sites should be shut down. Some believe in the need for free speech, and believe that these sites can be a springboard for further discussion with patients. I am on the side of those who would like to stop these websites, or at least counteract them with other sites offering accurate knowledge about eating disorders. These new sites could be run by healthcare professionals, interested teenagers, or even recovered patients. My reason for strongly opposing the sites is that they are not only seen by patients, they are also potentially seen by other impressionable children and teenagers. I worry that someone at risk for an eating disorder, who does not yet have good judgment, may be negatively influenced or harmed by them.

Effective Treatment Is Available

Despite the difficulties of treatment, effective treatment is available, and especially if begun early, can often lead to a cure, or at least a positive change in the life of a patient with an eating disorder. Most patients with eating disorders will need some form of medical monitoring as well as psychotherapy or counseling.

Who Provides Treatment?

Treatment may be provided by any or all of the following:

- Medical doctors.
- Psychiatrists.
- Psychologists.
- Social workers.
- Nurse practitioners.
- Nutritionists.

Treatment is usually best provided by a team of health care professionals who are knowledgeable in the care of patients with eating disorders. Many times the primary care doctor will coordinate the care. Before beginning treatment, the individual should have a thorough medical and mental assessment, and then treatment should be tailored to that person's needs. There is no one way to treat eating disorders.

Initial Assessment

The assessment, which may be done by one or more health care providers, should include a thorough history, a physical exam and the evaluation of lab tests.

HISTORY

Questions will be asked about medical and psychological, dietary, and any family history that may be relevant, as well as about food attitudes and weight and shape concerns.

PHYSICAL EXAM

The physical examination is done to determine vital signs and height, weight and body mass index, as well as to check for any underlying medical problems or medical complications.

LAB TESTS

A set of lab tests will be ordered or reviewed. These may vary depending on the diagnosis. The following tests are routinely done for most patients:

- Complete blood count.
- Blood chemistry and electrolyte studies (including magnesium and phosphorus levels in malnourished patients).
  - Liver function tests.
  - Cholesterol level.
  - Urinalysis.
  - Thyroid function tests.

The following tests are done in selected patients if needed:

- Blood tests: sedimentation rate, pregnancy test, hormone levels, amylase level.
  - Urine drug screen.
  - Electrocardiogram.
  - DEXA study to assess for osteoporosis.
  - Stool studies.
  - Other radiological studies, including Chest X-ray.
  - Echocardiogram.

Although lab tests can be very helpful, do not be falsely reassured by normal findings. Lab tests can be normal even if a patient is quite ill or malnourished.

Treatment Plan

After the initial assessment, a treatment plan will be made. A decision will also be made as to whether the person can safely be treated as an outpatient, or whether he or she is ill enough to require hospitalization or partial hospitalization.

MEDICAL MANAGEMENT AND MONITORING

After the initial assessment and physical exam, the patient should continue to be monitored by a medical doctor. This doctor can be part of an "eating disorder team" or in some cases can be the patient's primary care physician. Eating disorders can cause a number of medical problems and uncomfortable symptoms.

The medical doctor can monitor the patient's health, check for medical complications, and answer questions.

A psychiatrist is an important part of the team. Psychiatrists can prescribe medications for associated problems such as depression and anxiety, and are also able to provide therapy.

NUTRITIONAL COUNSELING

A dietician or nutritionist gives education about nutritional needs and can help the patient develop a normal and healthy eating plan. Ideally a registered dietician with expertise in the field of eating disorders will assess for nutritional deficiencies, provide guidance concerning meal planning, and teach the individual and family about healthy nutrition. Together with the patient the dietician can help create meal plans that are tolerable and acceptable. Food journals are often used to record daily food intake and exercise. These can also be used to write down emotions related to food and eating.

Although many patients do have some knowledge about nutrition, further education about the importance of healthy nutrition and the dangers of restriction can be valuable. If you are receiving nutritional counseling, you should be able to ask the dietician questions you may have about foods and calories and weight, but remember that most dieticians are not therapists. Your therapist will be the one to deal with more personal and emotional issues.

Nutritional counseling has several goals for the patient:

- To achieve a healthy weight.
- To become accepting of that weight.
- To be able to eat balanced meals and snacks when hungry, without the fear of getting fat.
- To be able to stop eating when full.
- To live without obsessions about food or weight.
- To stop dangerous behaviors such as bingeing, purging, excessive exercise and dieting.
- To become knowledgeable about nutritional requirements.

PSYCHOTHERAPY

Among the possibilities are individual therapy, family therapy, and group therapy.

Individual Therapy

Individual therapy can take various forms. One possibility is *cognitive behavioral therapy (CBT)*. The concept behind this therapy is that we can change negative behaviors by changing our way of thinking. Cognitive behavioral therapy has been shown to be quite effective for people with bulimia nervosa. This treatment also leads to better understanding of one's own behaviors, which can lead to learning alternative, healthier behaviors. CBT is hard work and is usually better for older, motivated teenagers.

Important components of CBT are:

- Self-monitoring.
- Meal planning.
- Understanding triggers and consequences of bingeing or starving oneself.
- Restructuring one's thinking.
- Preventing relapse.

Another type of therapy is *interpersonal therapy*, which has also been found to have some success in treating people with bulimia or binge-eating disorder. The idea is that the treatment and outcome are influenced by interpersonal relationships between the patient and significant others. The treatment is aimed at helping the person deal better with interpersonal problems. An example is the problem of separation, for example when a young person moves away from home to begin college.

Treatment is divided into three phases. In the first phase, the problem areas are identified, including possible interpersonal triggers of binge eating. In the second phase, possible solutions to problems are identified, with the person trying to implement these solutions. In the third phase, progress is assessed. The patient and her health care providers work on issues related to prevention and relapse.

Some people, especially teenagers or young adults with eating disorders of recent onset, do well with short-term therapy. However, others with more chronic eating disorders may require more long-term treatment, which may involve psychodynamic approaches focusing on the patient's inner world. Treatment may take several years.

Family Therapy

Family therapy is an important part of the treatment of young people with eating disorders. It is especially effective in the case of teenagers with anorexia nervosa of short duration. An eating disorder should be considered a problem of the whole family, not only of the individual suffering with the eating disorder. The illness usually impacts all members of the family, especially when the young person is still living at home.

Important goals of family therapy are:

- To identify any areas of stress in the family.
- To find healthy ways to deal with stress.
- To improve communication.
- To improve trust.
- To identify roles among family members.

Blame is not useful. There are many factors that play a part in causing someone to have an eating disorder. Family stress can precipitate an eating disorder, but it can also *result* from someone having an eating disorder. Any stress affecting one family member will have a ripple effect on the other family members. Parents and siblings can often play a big role in helping someone get better. They can also help the therapist get a better understanding of family problems.

Janice was sixteen years old when her pediatrician diagnosed her with anorexia nervosa. She was brought into the office by her mother, who herself was still struggling with an eating disorder. In spite of Janice's low weight, she was brought to her doctor because her menstrual cycle had stopped, rather than because of the weight loss. After calculating Janice's ideal body weight, the doctor explained that her weight and body fat were extremely low, which was the reason for the absence of her menstrual cycle. He recommended beginning a nutritional program to regain weight, as well as a referral to a therapist.

Janice's mother voiced her concerns about her daughter gaining too much weight. She felt that Janice looked good as she was, and she believed that her daughter felt better about herself when she was thin. In this family there was a very high value placed on appearance, and a lot of pressure to look a certain way, which included being thin. As Janice lost weight, she received positive reinforcement from everyone around her, and this only strengthened her resolve to diet. Treatment focused on involving the whole family and educating them about eating disorders and their dangers. Both individual and family therapy were begun.

Group Therapy

Group therapy can help as it allows patients to share feelings with others in a similar situation. It also reminds them that they are not alone. Groups are usually less costly than individual therapy, as one or two health care providers can see a number of people in one session. "Group therapy" refers to *therapeutic or treatment groups*, which should not be confused with support groups. Groups of patients meet for a number of sessions, and are guided by a health professional.

Group members can:

- Talk about their experiences in a safe setting.
- Explore ways of dealing with different situations.
- Learn to interact and be comfortable with others.
- Learn to share feelings and express emotions.

Not everyone will be a candidate for group therapy. Some patients may be too ill to function well in this setting.

Individual and Family Education

Each visit to a health care provider can be an opportunity to learn more about eating disorders, as well as how they affect the people around you.

Medication

The main form of treatment for people suffering with eating disorders is a form of psychotherapy. On the other hand, medications are often used, either to treat associated problems such as depression, obsessive-compulsive symptoms or anxiety, or to help regulate eating and prevent relapse. Patients and parents are sometimes worried about starting a medication such as an antidepressant for eating disorders. They may be concerned that the medication will alter their personality, or they may worry that they will become addicted. Neither of these is usually a problem. However, medications should not take the place of counseling.

Other Forms of Therapy

There are several other possibilities for therapy, usually in combination with the therapies mentioned above. They include:

- Movement therapy.
- Body image therapy.
- Stress management.
- Relaxation techniques.

Where Are Patients Treated?

Outpatient Treatment

Most people with eating disorders can be treated in an outpatient setting, with regular follow-up. They are able to continue with their normal routines. Someone with mild eating problems may only need to follow up every two weeks, but a person with a very low body weight, or someone who is throwing up daily, may need follow-up as often as twice a week or more.

One of the following levels of hospital-based treatment becomes necessary when medical, psychological or behavioral problems become more severe.

INPATIENT TREATMENT

Inpatient hospitalization is considered in certain situations, including:

- Severe or rapid weight loss.
- Severe medical complications such as irregular heart rate or electrolyte abnormalities.
- Severe psychiatric complications or associated disorders.
- Significant medical illnesses such as diabetes.
- Indications that the person is suicidal or homicidal.
- Other dangerous behavior including running away.
- Unsuccessful outpatient treatment.

Most inpatient and day hospital eating disorder treatment programs use a team approach. Medical doctors, psychiatrists, therapists and nutritionists are usually all part of the team. Patients usually eat supervised meals together, and have the opportunity to participate in classes as well as various forms of therapy.

Patients do better when their discharge weight is as close as possible to ideal body weight, and not too low.

DAY HOSPITAL TREATMENT

The person spends all day in the day hospital program, but returns home at night to sleep.

This program gives patients a structured environment and is a cheaper alternative to inpatient treatment for patients who are ill but don't require full hospitalization. It can be useful in the following circumstances:

• As a step-down after hospitalization, before continuing outpatient treatment.

• When a patient has not responded to outpatient treatment, but is not sick enough to need full hospitalization.

• When regular supervision, including supervised meals, is required.

• When the person needs daily or frequent monitoring or lab testing.

RESIDENTIAL CARE

Residential care is considered for patients who need long-term treatment. Treatment may last as long as several weeks or months. The longer stay allows them to stabilize their eating patterns, and gives them more time to address underlying issues. They receive less monitoring and supervision than they would in an inpatient setting. Patients may transfer to a residential center after being discharged from an inpatient unit.

Let's Review the Goals of Treatment

• To restore and maintain a healthy weight.
• To receive treatment for medical complications.
• To receive treatment for associated conditions.
• To stop dangerous behaviors such as bingeing and purging.
• To develop a healthy relationship with food.
• To develop healthy levels of activity.
• To improve self-esteem.
• To improve mood.
• To improve relationships.
• To learn healthy ways to deal with stress.
• To develop healthy goals unrelated to food or weight.
• To prevent complications and achieve long-term remission/ recovery.

These are all realistic goals!

Treatment for Specific Conditions

Treatment can make many patients very anxious, as the very thing most of them fear is gaining weight. I've heard some people with eating disorders express fear that everyone will notice if they gain even a pound. Others have worried that if they gain a pound, they will lose all control, and keep gaining weight until they become fat. As patients start to become well, however, the anxiety lessens.

ANOREXIA NERVOSA

Nutritional Consultation

A target weight should be set for any patient who is significantly underweight. If a person eats less than his or her body requires, the body won't get what it needs for normal metabolism and adequate growth and body repair. Also, when a person is malnourished, the brain doesn't function as well, and thinking is impaired. Before effective therapy can begin, weight should be regained.

A nutritional counselor or other health care provider should assess the amount of physical activity, particularly if it seems excessive, as this will increase calorie requirement and can put an underweight person at increased risk. In general, a person who is medically unstable or significantly underweight should not participate in physical activity.

Anorexic patients who are treated outside of the hospital should initially be expected to gain about one or two pounds per week. Sicker patients are hospitalized. In the hospital weight is gained more quickly, and meals and daily calorie intake can be planned under the guidance of a registered dietician. Patients should be monitored closely during this stage to make sure they do not develop complications such as fluid overload or electrolyte imbalances. It is important that the patient and family receive ongoing nutritional counseling and education.

Nutritional counseling will also look at whether a person feels or responds to hunger signals. If you have an eating disorder, you may not at first be able to rely on your own hunger signals to tell you when you want to eat and when you are satisfied. You will probably need to rely on the dietician to plan your meals with you initially.

Psychotherapy

The therapist must address the symptoms as well as the issues that contributed to the eating disorder. Psychotherapy is more effective once the patient has started gaining weight. Patients may respond to individual, group, or family therapy, or a combination of the above. Because anorexia nervosa is a chronic illness, ongoing psychotherapy is usually required for at least a year, and sometimes may take as long as five years.

Anorexia nervosa is a difficult illness to treat, but involving the family in the treatment of teenagers with anorexia nervosa has been shown to be of great benefit for many patients. The goal is to work on improving family relationships and to increase understanding of the eating disorder and how it may affect the members of the family. The therapist also teaches family members ways to cope with difficult feelings and situations that may arise. Family therapy is especially successful for a young person with anorexia nervosa if begun early on in the illness. Engagement of the family in treatment and commitment to therapy are important factors in affecting treatment outcome.

Medication

Medication is not the primary treatment for people with anorexia nervosa. A combination of restoring nutrition and psychotherapy or counseling is more effective. However, drugs may be used to treat associated problems, such as depression, anxiety or obsessive-compulsive symptoms. They are also sometimes used to prevent relapse amongst patients who have regained their weight. Sometimes medications are also used to treat gastrointestinal symptoms that often occur in people with anorexia nervosa.

Bulimia Nervosa

The main goal is to decrease or eliminate binge eating and purging behaviors and to establish a normal pattern of eating. Unrealistic assessments of weight and shape, perfectionism and low self-esteem also need to be addressed. Treatments include nutritional consultation and meal planning, psychotherapy, and medications when appropriate.

Nutritional Counseling

It is important to develop a pattern of eating regular, non-binge meals, and to try to avoid going for longer than four hours without eating. Eating regularly lessens the chance of excessive hunger, food obsessing, and bingeing. Research also shows that a structured pattern of eating lessens the negative feelings about food and eating.

Nutritional counseling is also important to increase the variety of foods eaten, to decrease behaviors such as skipping meals, and to encourage healthy but not excessive exercising. This is important even in the case of patients who are within a normal weight range.

Psychotherapy

The psychotherapy method of choice depends on the person's development, associated conditions, family situation, and preference, among other things.

Cognitive behavioral therapy, which involves changing negative behaviors by changing our way of thinking, has been shown to be very effective in the treatment of bulimia nervosa. It also deals with understanding one's behaviors and learning new behavior patterns, and involves self-monitoring. It was originally introduced in the late 1970s, but has only been used to treat people with bulimia since 1981. In the case of bulimia, cognitive behavioral therapy addresses the problem behaviors of bingeing and purging and replaces them with a normal eating pattern. It also challenges the abnormal perceptions about body shape and weight. Treatment usually lasts about twenty weeks.

Interpersonal psychotherapy can also be very useful in treating people with bulimia or binge eating. Family therapy should be considered whenever appropriate, but especially when teenagers are still living with their parents. Finally, some patients respond well to group therapy.

Medication

Medications can be effective as one component of the therapy of bulimia. They can be used to treat symptoms such as depression or anxiety, to reduce the urge to binge, or to prevent relapse. Fluoxetine (Prozac) is the drug which has been most studied in the treatment of bulimia nervosa.

Many patients do best with a combination of cognitive behavioral therapy and medication.

TREATMENT FOR BINGE-EATING DISORDER

Treatment should involve establishing normal healthy eating patterns and encouraging a safe and healthy exercise routine. The goal is also to improve body image and self-esteem. Binge-eating disorder is usually treated with some form of psychotherapy, such as behavior therapy or cognitive behavioral therapy. Medications such as antidepressants may sometimes be used together with therapy to treat depression and to lessen the frequency of bingeing and the preoccupation with food.

Finding Help

HOW TO FIND AN EATING DISORDER CENTER

- Ask your primary care physician.
- Ask a school counselor.
- Ask a hospital in the area.
- Ask a recovered patient.
- Contact one of the eating disorder associations, which often provide referrals.
- Check in your local telephone book or on the internet. (See this book's Appendix for a list of resources.)

HOW TO FIND A THERAPIST

Finding the right therapist can be one of the keys to a successful outcome. You should choose a therapist who has experience in working with eating disorders, and someone with whom you feel comfortable speaking.

Here are some ways to locate a therapist:

- Ask for a referral from your primary care physician or psychiatrist.
- Ask for a referral from the nearest teaching hospital or an eating disorder center.

- Ask friends or recovered patients. Hearing about someone from families who are happy with care can go a long way to making you feel more comfortable.
- Try an eating disorders referral center. (See this book's Appendix for a list of resources.)
- Look in the telephone book.

When you get the name of a therapist, you should obtain certain information:

- Check on the license and credentials of the therapist, who will usually have a Ph.D. or be a licensed clinical social worker.
- Find out how long the therapist has been treating eating disorders.
- Find out if treatment will be reimbursed by insurance, and if not, what your options are.

It may be worthwhile to schedule a meeting with the therapist to discuss philosophies of treatment.

Moving Forward: Through Treatment and Beyond

Once in treatment, patients need to rebuild their self-esteem, regain control over their lives, and set new goals.

I don't think people with eating disorders are completely cured until they have addressed their abnormal perceptions of weight and shape and replaced unhealthy beliefs, goals and values with healthy ones. Even if they stop bingeing and purging, they may still struggle daily with low self-esteem and other issues relating to self-worth. These problems need to be addressed.

Young people should be guided to develop healthy self-esteem and to take pride in their accomplishments unrelated to appearance. They will once again learn the satisfaction of doing well in school, being creative, helping someone in need, or being a good friend.

Laura's Story

Laura, who seemed to outsiders to be almost perfect at everything, developed anorexia nervosa at the age of sixteen. Prior to developing the eating disorder, she had been getting straight A's in school, was on the debating team and was the most popular girl in her class. Her grandmother became very ill, and this put a great emotional strain on the whole family. Her schedule was disrupted and her grades slipped to B's and a C. She worried about her parents and became overwhelmed by everything, including issues in the local and national news. She felt helpless. She began dieting and found that in this arena she had some control. Unfortunately she went too far, until soon her eating disorder consumed her life.

Laura wanted to be perfect, and she thought she could achieve perfection if she became thin enough. She now knows that her goals were unrealistic and didn't lead to happiness or success. No one can be perfect. Young people need to know that their best *is* good enough—for themselves, their family and friends, and society.

Angela, Katie and Sarah's Story

Angela, Katie and Sarah were inpatients in the eating disorder center of a hospital. They identified with each other immediately and referred to themselves as "the anorexics."

When I asked Angela to describe herself, it was difficult for her to see past her eating disorder. That was her life and her goal, and that was what took up every ounce of her energy.

Katie, by her own admission, was referred to by her parents and friends as "the one who doesn't eat." That was her identity, and she believed that if that identity were to be taken away, she would be lost.

It can take a long time for patients with eating disorders to appreciate the other part of their personalities—their strengths and their talents. But when they do, they often discover a new and wonderful life. As Sarah became well, she began seeing herself as a good student, an artist and a good daughter. She began taking pride in those attributes and slowly started realizing that she would be accepted by others whether she was thin or not.

Eating disorders and their associated conditions can cause serious harm, both mental and physical. No matter how "good" someone with an eating disorder appears, or whether they still seem to be able to function, these conditions cannot be ignored. One young lady told me that if she had an eating disorder, so did many of her college friends. Maybe they do. That doesn't make it acceptable or less dangerous. Fortunately, treatment is available.

If you think you may have an eating disorder, get professional help as soon as possible.

- Speak to your parents or a trusted family member.
- Go to your primary care physician for an assessment and referral if needed.
- Be evaluated at an eating disorder center, if appropriate.
- Become educated about eating disorders and their complications.
- Be hopeful about your recovery.

Future Research

To improve outcomes, continuous research is being done on the effectiveness of medications as well as various forms of therapy used to treat eating disorders.

Because studies suggest that eating disorders are inherited, scientists are searching for genes that might make a person susceptible to developing an eating disorder. Discovery of a related gene or genes will allow for better understanding of eating disorders and the development of better treatments.

10

Recovery

So often I am asked whether patients with eating disorders can recover fully. The answer is yes. While not everyone suffering from an eating disorder recovers completely, if a person is motivated to get well, puts in the effort and gets appropriate professional treatment, the chances of recovery are very high.

Many people with eating disorders, particularly anorexia nervosa, are very ambivalent about getting well. Getting well means that they have to face the very thing they fear most—gaining weight.

Personal Stories

ELAINE'S STORY

For many years, Elaine, an eighteen-year-old woman with anorexia nervosa and purging, moved from one therapist to another, almost as though she were looking for someone who would tell her what she wanted to hear. What they all told her, however, was that she was very ill and needed to gain weight, possibly to be hospitalized. As much as Elaine disliked living with her illness, she hated even more the thought of being hospitalized and having to gain weight, so she didn't follow the recommendations given to her.

One day she was watching a television program about a patient who died of a heart complication because of an eating disorder. Something inside her changed. It was not that she had never heard about the dangers of anorexia nervosa, but this story hit home. That very day she made a call to one last eating disorder treatment group. She made up her mind that she was not going to die. She decided that she was going to get well, and she did.

Elaine was hospitalized for a prolonged period and then continued with intensive outpatient treatment. She is now married with a child of her own, and is finally free from the illness that kept her from living her life.

Read what some patients had to say about their recoveries:

CHERYL'S STORY

Cheryl is a twenty-six-year-old mother of two young girls. She was hospitalized three times before the age of 18, and missed many months of school and years of having fun with friends. When she looks back on her life with anorexia nervosa, she can hardly believe that she is the same person. "I wasn't a fun person. My world revolved around food and my illness. I had no time for friends or even my family."

I asked her what turned things around.

"I decided that I had to get well. I could not continue this way any longer. I was lucky to have a very supportive family that would not give up on me. Group therapy and becoming more involved in my community also helped a lot. The community involvement helped me forget about myself for a while and help others instead. This made me feel fulfilled and helped a lot with my self-esteem. Believe me, the poor and homeless didn't care what I looked like."

ALLISON'S STORY

Allison, the young administrative assistant I wrote about earlier, is doing better, but still struggles with weight and food issues. She says: "Everything revolves around food. At work, all people talk about is how they want to lose weight, or they talk about what they are having for lunch. We're going on a work picnic on Sunday, and I'm already worried about what I'll eat, and how I'm going to have to eat in front of all those people. When I visit my family the conversation revolves around how everyone looks, and whether they have lost or gained weight. I can't get away from it. I feel that if I don't look a certain way, I won't be good enough for them."

Emily's Story

Emily has recovered from anorexia nervosa and is now a happily married mother of a two-year-old son. She was very kind to share her story.

In high school, Emily always had mild weight and body image concerns and attempted several diets without much success. Serious symptoms of an eating disorder really began when she turned seventeen and left home for college in another city. Although she was a high achiever and a popular student, the separation from her home and family and the change in lifestyle seemed overwhelming to Emily. Dancing became her comfort, and she found that restricting foods helped her maintain her lower weight and gave her a sense of being in control.

Towards the end of her freshman year, her colleagues were stunned by her weight loss, but not one of them felt comfortable approaching her with their concerns. She rarely saw her parents, as home was many miles away, but on the rare occasions that she did, she told them her weight loss resulted from dancing and the stress of studying.

About that time, Emily began dating a young man in medical school. It became very clear to him that she was suffering from anorexia nervosa. In spite of their difficult relationship as Emily became more withdrawn because of her illness, he loved her and was determined to help. After several attempts, he persuaded her to get help from a physician who specialized in eating disorders.

Emily went reluctantly, although she then understood that she was in serious need of help. Although she was on the right path, it took several years of counseling before she really felt that she could live life without constantly fearing and obsessing about food and her weight.

I asked her what had helped her most. "Having the support of someone who really cared about me and would not give up on me," she answered.

Emily is not completely free of weight concerns. She still monitors what she eats to a point, although she is no longer hard on herself if she eats a little more than usual, or skips her workouts for a day or two.

She enjoys her family tremendously, and believes that the best gift she can give her son is to help him develop good self-esteem, something she didn't have until recently.

What Are the Chances of Recovering?

In general, with treatment, the outcome for most people with eating disorders is good, although complete recovery can take many years. A certain percentage of individuals do continue to have mild symptoms, and some do develop chronic eating disorders that don't respond to treatment, but with appropriate treatment most people get better. Some patients with anorexia nervosa go on to develop bulimia (or, more rarely, vice versa).

We should always take eating disorders very seriously. The mortality rate for patients with anorexia nervosa is much higher than that of the general population in that age group. Among patients with bulimia, although the risk is higher than in the non-eating disorder population, the mortality rate is low.

People who have recovered from anorexia nervosa tend to be thin, and some still have some of the features of anorexia, e.g. perfectionistic attitudes or a desire for thinness. Those who have recovered from bulimia may still have concerns about their weight or shape, and may have a tendency to either restrict foods, or to overeat.

What Is Recovery?

Recovery is more than maintaining a safe weight and being free from medical complications. True recovery has occurred when you are free from constant thoughts or obsessions about eating, food and weight. It occurs when you begin to have control over your life and when you can once again take pleasure in everyday activities, friendships and relationships. This does not mean that you won't have occasional self-doubts, or concerns about food and weight issues, as many healthy people do, but they will be fleeting, and will not interfere with your life.

After reaching initial treatment goals, most patients need to be monitored for at least a couple of years, with the goal and expectation of being cured. Reaching your ideal body weight is only the beginning of treatment. The ultimate goal is to increase your self-esteem, change your belief system so that you no longer place such a high value on appearance and thinness, and find healthier ways of dealing with stress.

How Does Recovery Begin?

To begin the recovery process you must:

- Accept that there is a problem.
- Accept that you need help.
- Want to get well.
- Be prepared to take risks.
- Talk to a parent or trusted adult about your problem to the extent that you are able.
- Get help from a professional or team of professionals with experience in the treatment of eating disorders.

Once you have recognized your eating disorder and have asked for help, you have begun the process of recovery. The next stage requires a real willingness to change your life and continue the process of becoming well. Allow yourself to accept help. Remember that you (perhaps together with your family) are making the choice to have treatment. Recovery can be difficult and can take time, especially if the eating disorder is longstanding, so be patient.

An important part of recovery is learning to *restructure your thinking*. You will learn to challenge your beliefs and challenge the media. Most importantly, you will learn to think about yourself in a positive way.

Challenge Your Beliefs

Once your weight is in a healthy range, and you are beginning the process of recovery, it is important to challenge some of your beliefs and thoughts about food and weight. Some examples of these false beliefs that are so intrusive are:

- Foods are either good or bad.
- If I gain any weight, I will become fat.
- All fat is bad.
- If I gain one pound, everyone will notice.
- If I eat more, I will lose all control.

CHALLENGE THE MEDIA

Stay away from magazines that only portray very thin models. Challenge cultural stereotypes. Don't tolerate prejudice on the basis of size or physical appearance. Accept yourself as well as other people for who they really are.

THINK ABOUT YOURSELF IN A POSITIVE WAY

It's important to remind yourself that it is not your size but your character that makes you a good person. Instead of being overly critical of yourself, remember your good attributes. Learn to love the fact that you are different from anyone else. Learn to appreciate your body and the way it is uniquely you.

When things get tough, you can:

- Remind yourself of why you want to get well.
- Think about family members that love you.
- Remember the friends that care about you.
- Consider that perhaps there is someone you could help in the future.
- Remember that no matter how hard you have been on yourself, you do matter, and you can make a difference.
- Remember that you too have the opportunity to set goals and achieve your dreams.

Lapses

It's not unusual for people recovering from eating disorders to have occasional lapses, such as restricting their food intake for a day, or exercising too much for a day or two. If this happens, try to take the time to see why you "slipped." This is not the same as a relapse, and should be used as a learning experience.

Relapse

Many people who have recovered from an eating disorder worry about whether their eating disorder will return. It is impossible to say for certain that it won't. On the other hand, most people do recover from eating disorders, and if symptoms do return, they can be treated. A good therapist will help you deal with issues that may come up after recovery and will prepare you to deal with challenging situations. It's good for you to have a plan ready in case of relapse.

What are some of the warning signs of a lapse or relapse?

- Dieting
- Skipping meals
- Cutting out all fats
- Excessive exercising
- Becoming preoccupied with food, calories and weight issues
- Weighing yourself every day
- Binge eating
- Purging
- Feeling shame or guilt after eating
- Feeling lonely and depressed

If you notice any of these symptoms returning, speak to your doctor or therapist as soon as possible.

The following can help prevent a relapse:

- A strong motivation to get well.
- A good support system—family and friends.

- Keeping in touch with a counselor or therapist.
- Having resources or a support group available.
- Having a clear plan of action in case of a lapse.
- Keeping in perspective the negative and harmful effects of dieting and the eating disorder.
- Learning ways of coping with stress, such as taking a walk, drawing, or calling a friend.
- Recording activities in a journal.
- Having a satisfying job.
- Engaging in enjoyable hobbies.
- Helping someone in need or doing charity work.
- Setting goals for the future.

Support Groups

Many patients recovering from eating disorders find support groups very helpful. Ask your doctor or therapist for a recommendation. People with eating disorders are often socially isolated, so it can be very helpful and comforting to connect with others with whom you can share your feeling and thoughts. Support groups are not the same as treatment groups as no therapy is provided. People in various stages of recovery can support each other during these informal sessions. Support groups should not take the place of therapy.

Family Support

ANITA'S STORY

Anita was diagnosed with anorexia nervosa after she left home for college. She was a high achiever, had a loving family, and grew up in a good home environment. There was a strong family history of depression, and Anita herself was treated with antidepressants for mild depression. To everyone else, she "had it all together," but to Anita, she was never good enough. When she began college, her self-esteem was very low, and she began dieting. Many of her friends were dieting too, but when they stopped dieting, she continued. During one of her visits home, she appeared so ill that she was taken to the hospital. She had a very difficult year, requiring weekly therapy and two emergency room visits, but luckily Anita is finally on the road to recovery.

"It's so difficult," she told me. "The thing that's getting me through this, is that I know my mom and dad are there for me." It was true. Both her parents stood by her through the good times and the bad. She knew that they loved her even when she was not sure that she loved herself, and that was what she needed most.

MICHELLE'S STORY

Since the age of ten, Michelle had a history of body image problems and engaging in dieting behaviors. When she was fourteen years old, she started another diet, and this time lost an excessive amount of weight. She was taken to her family doctor and was diagnosed as having anorexia nervosa.

Her family situation was not easy. She was an only child and her parents were on the brink of a divorce. Her father, an attorney, worked long hours and often returned home after she was asleep. Her mother did the best she could, but the family stresses took a toll on her.

When Michelle's parents became aware of her illness and the diagnosis of anorexia nervosa was confirmed, they understood that in order to give her the best chance of recovery, they had to work together. It was recommended that both parents participate in family therapy. Even though this was difficult for her parents because of their strained relationship, they were determined that they would do whatever it took to help their daughter. Her dad decreased his work hours so that he could attend weekly family meetings, and her mom attended those meetings and also took her to her other therapy and nutrition sessions.

It was a difficult year, with ups and downs, but it finally seemed to pay off. Michelle started improving steadily, and in addition, her parents started communicating better to the point where both now seem confident that they will make their marriage work.

I believe that parent involvement and support is a very important part of the treatment and recovery process. Young people with involved, caring parents have a big advantage. In certain circumstances this is not an option, however. Some families cannot be involved. They may be too far away, emotionally incapable, or too controlling, among other things. If you do live with your parents, and they are loving and supportive, talk to them about your feelings and your goals. Help them become knowledgeable about eating disorders. Explore various resources and avenues of support together.

Prognosis

When someone is treated for an eating disorder, the goal of treatment of course is to achieve full recovery. The time to recovery can be relatively short for someone with a mild eating disorder, or it can take many years for someone more ill. Although full recovery is possible, unfortunately, it is not always the case. Some patients continue with a chronic course. However, even when recovery is not full, treatment can greatly improve someone's quality of life.

11

Prevention

We live in a culture that is obsessed with outward appearance and the achievement of certain physical ideals. These ideals are often unrealistic and include extreme thinness for women and muscularity for men. Desire for these ideals is strengthened by images seen in magazines and on television, and messages that glorify thinness and persuade us to spend lots of time and money to achieve beauty and happiness. Young people who try to achieve such unrealistic ideals may diet or engage in unhealthy eating patterns and develop eating disorders and associated problems. In addition to the young men and women who suffer from eating disorders or related conditions, many more have significant body image concerns.

Treating the millions of people suffering with eating disorders is an enormous task, and success is not inevitable. The only long-term solution is preventing eating disorders from occurring in the first place. Prevention must take place on every level. The individual, the family and society must all get involved.

What Can an Individual Do?

You can do many things as an individual—for yourself and for people you care about. You can:

- Learn about eating disorders.
- Watch for warning signs in yourself or others.
- Be cautious about dieting.
- Eat regular balanced meals.
- Exercise in moderation.
- Learn how to handle stress in healthy ways.
- Like yourself for who you are inside rather than for your appearance and size.
- Set goals for your future.
- Remind yourself regularly about what's really important in life.
- Challenge the media messages about thinness and appearance. Become a critical viewer.
- Don't tolerate stereotyping on the basis of appearance or size.

Learn About Eating Disorders

It is important to learn whatever you can about eating disorders and their harmful effects. Learn how to evaluate our society's messages about thinness in a critical way. Understand that becoming thin will not automatically make you happy or successful. There are many ways in which you can become more knowledgeable about eating disorders. Your physician will be able to give you a list of resources and reading material. Resources are also listed in the Appendix at the back of this book, and reading material is listed in the Bibliography.

Take Note of Warning Signs

If warning signs are seen in a person at risk, early action might prevent an eating disorder. Eating disorders are more easily prevented than cured, and the earlier they are diagnosed and appropriately treated, the better the outcome. If you think you have an eating disorder or you are preoccupied with thoughts about food and your weight, or engaging in dangerous behaviors related to eating, speak to your parents or a trusted family member and get professional help as soon as possible.

When Does "Trying to Lose Weight" Become a Problem?

Most people have concerns about their bodies at some time or another. They may wish for a flatter abdomen, thinner thighs, or less flabby arms. To try to achieve their goals, they may exercise longer, or even cut down on calories for a short period of time. However, their dissatisfaction remains in perspective, and they are still able to continue with their lives in a normal way. It is when the concern about their appearance, food and weight becomes an obsession, interferes with their lives, and stands in the way of happiness, that an eating disorder exists.

Be Cautious About Dieting

When I say "dieting," I am referring to significantly restricting or limiting the intake of food and calories in order to lose weight. Do you know that about 40 to 50 percent of American women are trying to lose weight at any point in time? But uncontrolled dieting can have dangerous consequences, and can put a vulnerable person at risk for developing an eating disorder.

Not everyone who diets develops an eating disorder, but eating disorders almost always begin with a diet. Not only can uncontrolled dieting cause nutritional imbalances, but it can set you up for hunger which in turn puts you at risk for binge eating. Think back to a time when perhaps you have deprived yourself of certain "forbidden" foods for a while. Eventually you begin to crave that food. When you restrict food and calories for a long time, it is a normal response to become preoccupied by food. On the other hand, when you develop a regular pattern of eating a balanced diet, the cravings and preoccupations with food disappear.

Instead of dieting, a nutritionist can help you develop a balanced meal plan consisting of all the nutrients your body needs. If you find that you turn to food instead of dealing with your feelings, try to find better ways of coping with strong feelings. If you are unable to do so, a counselor can help.

Unfortunately, many of your friends are probably dieting or talking about losing weight, and there is enormous pressure to join the crowd. I recently asked a tenth-grader if many of her friends were engaged in dieting behaviors, and she replied: "Pretty much my whole grade." Well, that may be an overstatement, but it is true that the number of girls trying to become thinner is very high. The percentage of boys trying to change their weight or shape is very significant too.

EAT REGULAR BALANCED MEALS

For the reasons we have discussed before, diets are not the answer to becoming healthier. One can eat regularly, without feeling hungry, and still remain healthy and avoid becoming overweight. Children and teenagers need enough calories and fats to grow and develop normally, and the amounts vary depending on age, sex, weight and activity level. You may ask your doctor or a dietician to help you determine your specific requirements.

Here are some nutrition tips:

• Eat three meals and one or two snacks every day and try not to go for longer than three to four hours without eating. This will help to keep you satisfied and prevent hunger and bingeing.

• Eat a healthy breakfast to provide you with energy and keep you alert.

• Make sure you eat a variety of foods from all the basic food groups, and get adequate amounts of proteins, fats and carbohydrates in your diet. Try to eat enough complex carbohydrates, such as whole grain breads and cereals, rather than white breads and white flour products.

• Try to eat at least 5 servings of fruits and vegetables every day. These provide vitamins and minerals, and are a good source of fiber. Experiment with different types of fruits and vegetables.

• Besides eating fruits and vegetables, you can also increase your intake of fiber by eating whole grains, beans and peas.

• Choose fluids such as water and fruit juices rather than sodas whenever possible.

• Have healthy snacks available in case you are hungry between meals. Examples of healthy snacks are yogurts, cut-up fruits and vegetables, air-popped popcorn, or whole wheat bread.

EXERCISE IN MODERATION

About thirty to sixty minutes of physical activity approximately five days a week is a healthy amount of exercise for most young people. You can be fit and feel good about yourself without becoming a renowned athlete. Choose an activity you enjoy, such as walking, biking or running. You could also put more activity into your daily routine, for example, by walking to the bus stop, or taking the stairs instead of the elevator. If you are exercising for several hours a day and are not training for the Olympics, you should ask yourself whether this could be part of an eating disorder.

LEARN HOW TO HANDLE STRESS

It has been shown that happy people don't necessarily have less stress, but are better able to deal with stress. People who are able to cope with stress, disappointment and life's inevitable setbacks in healthy ways seem to do much better.

Here are some ways to cope with stress:

• It helps to have a good support system—family and friends you can talk to.
• Learn relaxation techniques. Some people find that yoga helps, others relax in a warm bath.
• Take up an interesting new hobby such as art or photography. Doing something interesting and exciting can be distracting, and mastering a new hobby or skill can give a sense of accomplishment.
• Be flexible. Life deals us surprises sometimes. Try not to be too rigid.
• Have fun. People love to be around someone with a positive attitude.

If you are under excessive stress, feel very anxious or depressed, do ask for help from an adult family member, a counselor, or your physician. *Don't* turn to smoking, alcohol or drugs to solve your problems.

LIKE YOURSELF FOR WHO YOU ARE INSIDE

Self-esteem means feeling good about yourself and liking yourself, not only for the way you look, but for who you are inside. Good or positive self-esteem means that you like yourself all the time, not only when someone compliments you, or when you achieve a good grade at school. People with positive self-esteem are not as strongly influenced by what other people tell them to do, or by negative comments. Positive self-esteem gives them confidence and strength to believe in themselves. Respect yourself as a person. Ultimately you (not your friends) are the one who is responsible for making good decisions that will affect your life.

How can you develop a positive self-esteem?

- Accept yourself for who you are. No one is perfect.
- Do your very best, but don't be too hard on yourself if the outcome is not exactly what you expected. Be proud that you tried hard.
- Be realistic. It's okay to set high standards, but don't overdo it.
- Be proud of your achievements and successes.
- Trust yourself and your instincts. Nobody knows you better than you do.

SET GOALS FOR YOUR FUTURE

What is most important to you in life? Good health, family, friends, success? Ask yourself if being thin will help you achieve your goals. People with anorexia nervosa may experience short-lived feelings of achievement when they lose weight, but they constantly have to lose more weight to feel successful. In the end they never reach their goal, and their weight loss does not bring them happiness. Set goals for yourself that are not related to weight and appearance. Reward yourself for the small successes on the way.

REMEMBER WHAT'S REALLY IMPORTANT

I haven't seen two of my best friends for several years now, although we do keep in touch. One was a colleague of mine in medical school and the other a friend from high school. Unfortunately, because they live abroad, our paths haven't crossed for a long time. I think of them often. I remember how Amy and I had long discussions about school and friends and went sight-seeing together. Stephanie and I both studied music and enjoyed concerts. Most important of all, these were friends I could trust. I knew that if I asked them to do anything for me, they would, and vice versa. Never once when I think back to those times together do I dwell on how my friends looked. Never do I think, "I liked

Amy because she was tall and thin, or I liked Stephanie because she had long blonde hair."

Think to the future. What do you want to be remembered for? What will make you proud one day? My guess is that it will be your kindness and compassion, your accomplishments, or how you have contributed to helping people and our society.

WHAT CAN FAMILY MEMBERS DO?

Parents do have a significant effect on the development of their child's body image. Parental and family stress can contribute to or result from an eating disorder. Most parents of children with eating disorders are good people who are doing the best they can. Some parents may deny that there is a problem, or may feel guilty about somehow contributing to the problem. One mother broke down crying, asking her daughter for forgiveness, in case of anything she had said to contribute to her eating disorder.

The best thing a parent can do is to have their child evaluated and treated as soon as possible. Also, support from parents during the evaluation and treatment process seems to have a very positive effect. Because an eating disorder can affect all members of a family, parents and siblings may benefit from counseling and support too.

Parents should:

• Be cautious about perfectionism. They should praise their sons and daughters for their good efforts, even though the outcomes may not be perfect.

• Avoid criticizing each other or their children on appearance.

• Not tolerate teasing about weight or appearance.

• Acknowledge their children's successes unrelated to appearance.

• Emphasize the importance of health and fitness rather than thinness.

• Eat nutritious foods, instead of dieting, and participate in healthy exercise. Enjoy eating and make mealtimes pleasant. Parents should not obsess about food and calories.

If a child insists on going on a diet, the help of a nutritionist or a physician can be enlisted to create a healthy nutrition plan. Certain people are genetically predisposed to the development of an eating disorder, based on their personality type and their mood. If these vulnerable children express dislike of their bodies or the desire to diet, they should be watched very closely.

What Can Our Society Do?

- Increase community awareness of eating disorders.
- Increase education about the dangers of eating disorders.
- Promote community and school-based programs that encourage healthy attitudes about weight and eating.
- Promote responsible media.
- Educate children on effective life skills.
- Educate young people about challenging some of our cultural messages and viewing the media critically.
- Define the responsibilities of coaches and fitness instructors.

INCREASE COMMUNITY AWARENESS

To successfully prevent and treat eating disorders, communities need better understanding of these conditions. People need to realize that eating disorders are serious illnesses that can be life-threatening, and that they occur in both males and females. There is still too much misinformation regarding eating disorders. Lectures or discussion groups could be held regularly in schools, for example, to further promote awareness, and allow students to have their questions answered.

PROMOTE RESPONSIBLE MEDIA

We should all be aware that the images of super-thin models in the media are not realistic and do not portray a healthy ideal. The same is true for images of extremely muscular men. Constant exposure to these images can put young people at risk for engaging in unhealthy eating habits, excessive exercise, and even dangerous practices such as taking anabolic steroids. Advertising companies make a lot of money by encouraging people to buy beauty and diet products to make them better-looking. They have been quite successful, because the customer is buying their sales pitch and is buying the product. However, this eventually leads to disappointment, because in the end, being thin does not ensure happiness or popularity.

EDUCATE CHILDREN ON EFFECTIVE LIFE SKILLS

Young people who feel good about themselves and the way they look, and are able to cope with stress in a healthy way, are less likely to develop eating disorders. From a young age children should be taught effective life skills, such as ways to deal with stress, cope with disappointment, cultivate good relationships and develop high self-esteem. They should also be taught how to analyze the media critically and how to cope with pressures to become thin, as well as with teasing. Last, but not least, children should be encouraged to set healthy goals and to take pride in their accomplishments that are unrelated to appearance. These skills can be taught in school as well as at home, and can be incorporated into a curriculum from an early grade.

DEFINE THE RESPONSIBILITIES OF COACHES AND FITNESS INSTRUCTORS

Coaches and teachers have a strong influence on the body image of young people.

Here are two examples of the impact they can have.

A Positive Influence

Judy was a well-known dance instructor in a small town. Many young girls who dreamed of becoming dancers joined her classes. Meryl didn't look like the other girls, because she had always been overweight and they were so thin, but she loved to dance. Her mother had promised that she could join the group in her seventh grade, and so she did. Meryl struggled a bit at first—she wasn't used to doing so much exercise—but Judy encouraged her and praised her for her efforts, so she always felt as if she belonged. Meryl eventually became one of the group's best dancers. Most importantly, she danced because she loved dancing.

It was never about what she looked like. She was happy with who she was, and part of that was thanks to Judy.

A Negative Influence

Ann was a healthy young girl of average size who joined a gymnastics team when she was twelve. She was very fit and excelled at the floor exercise routines and the uneven bars. One day her instructor remarked that she could advance further if she were to lose a few pounds. The girl who had been so confident began to feel self-conscious. She started dieting, and continued dieting when she found that it was relatively easy to lose weight. Eventually she lost so much weight that she was unable to compete, and her gymnastics career was put on hold until her eating disorder was brought under control.

What Can Coaches and Instructors Do?

Coaches, physical education instructors and dance teachers should be cautious when working with their students and should recognize the unique health risks in athletes.

They should have some knowledge about the nutrition requirements of athletes and be able to recognize warning signs of eating disorders. They should also:

- Promote a healthy lifestyle.
- Be cautious about advising children or teenagers to lose weight.
- Discourage dangerous weight control methods.
- Be sensitive with respect to their attitudes and remarks to students, including those related to weight and appearance.
- Promote self-esteem in students.

As we have come to learn more about the causes of eating disorders, we are learning possible ways to prevent them. It will take effort on everyone's part—the individual, families, and our society. Because these illnesses are so serious, and because they affect not only every aspect of the sufferer's life but also the lives of the people around them, I think our efforts will be worthwhile.

12

Adolescent Obesity

There has been a great increase in the number of American children and teenagers who are overweight, and it is estimated that between one in four and one in five children in the United States is now obese or at risk for becoming obese. Obesity is now the most common nutritional disease among children in the United States. For this reason, prevention of obesity has become a major public health priority.

How Do We Define Obesity?

Weight alone is not an accurate measure of obesity or health. A better gauge is something called body mass index (BMI). This is calculated by dividing someone's weight in kilogram by their height in meters squared and is a standard measure used to assess obesity. It is an indicator of excess body fat and is quite simple to use.

Although there is an accepted range of normal for body mass index in *Adults*, there is no universal definition of obesity in children and teenagers. Normal body mass index varies with age for children and adolescents. A physician should be consulted to determine a child's proper BMI in relation to age and to determine if a child or adolescent is obese. A standard definition for obesity is a body mass index of greater or equal to 95 percent of normal for age and sex. Someone who falls between the 85th and 95th percentile is at risk for becoming obese.

Obesity is a serious problem. There are many medical and psychological complications and problems associated with obesity.

Medical Complications

Overweight teenagers have a higher risk of becoming overweight adults, and we know that being overweight as an adult sets a person up for the following serious health problems. Some of these problems are now being seen even in children and teenagers who are overweight.

DIABETES

Type 2 diabetes is usually associated with obesity. The number of children with Type 2 diabetes has risen dramatically in the last decade, and of those children, 85 percent are obese. Children at highest risk for developing Type 2 diabetes are those who are inactive, who overeat, and who have a family history of diabetes.

HIGH BLOOD PRESSURE

Obesity is a leading cause of high blood pressure in young people.

HIGH CHOLESTEROL

Obesity is associated with elevated cholesterol levels, and high cholesterol can increase a person's risk for heart disease.

HEART PROBLEMS

Being overweight puts added stress on the heart. This stress combined with high cholesterol can put even a young person at increased risk for heart disease.

Respiratory Problems

Being overweight can be associated with a serious condition called sleep apnea, in which a person stops breathing for a period of time during sleep. One of the symptoms of sleep apnea can be daytime sleepiness. Obesity can also aggravate symptoms of asthma.

Joints and Bones

Being overweight can put added stress on hips, knees, and other joints, increasing the risk of problems with these areas of the body. Because of the joint problems, people tend to exercise even less, and this becomes a vicious cycle.

Gallbladder Disease

Overweight adults are more likely to develop gallbladder disease and gallstones. This occurs in women more often than in men.

Menstrual Problems

Some menstrual problems are associated with being overweight. Also, young girls who are overweight often begin their menstrual cycle earlier.

Psychological Problems

Medical problems are not the only negative consequences of obesity in young people. Because our society places an extremely high value on fitness and thinness, teenagers who are overweight are frequently teased. As a result, overweight young people may feel shame, or may suffer from low self-esteem and develop social isolation. Sadly, there is still prejudice against people who are severely overweight. People are often stigmatized on the basis of appearance. They may have a more difficult time renting a house or apartment, getting a job and may even earn less money. Of course it's wrong for them to be treated this way, but it does happen.

It has been suggested that overweight people in general suffer more guilt and psychological problems because of their obesity. However, many studies do not find consistent differences with these problems when people who are overweight are compared to those who are not. It seems as if the effects of being overweight differ from person to person, so that some people may suffer serious psychological consequences, and others, few or none.

One common finding in people who are overweight is a negative body image. This can show up in the following ways:

- A preoccupation about their appearance.
- A belief that the way they look is tied to their self-worth.
- Social isolation.

What Do Teenagers Have to Say About Being Overweight?

Amanda, who is sixteen years old and has always been overweight, told me that she feels good about herself most of the time, and that she has friends who like her for who she is. She socializes quite a lot. She does not enjoy going shopping, however, especially shopping for clothes, as she feels bad about trying on clothes that often don't fit. She goes to movies with her friends, but rarely to the mall.

Nathan, who is fifteen, told me that he socializes with male friends, but feels very uncomfortable around girls because of his weight. When he compares himself to his more athletic friends, he feels that he doesn't measure up.

Several teenagers told me that they were teased, and that they wished people would not be judged on the basis of their appearance. Many told me that they pretended to make light of the teasing, and covered up the pain they felt inside.

Some teenagers wanted to lose weight because of health concerns. They had read about complications of obesity, and a few had a family history of obesity-related illnesses.

SHELLEY'S STORY

Shelley was a fourteen-year-old ninth-grader who was regularly teased at school. Because she was overweight, she was called all sorts of terrible names. Her defense mechanism was to act as if she didn't care at all, although the teasing caused her a lot of pain and affected her self-esteem. There was only one friend who really understood what she was going through, and that friend stood by her throughout that difficult year. The two began an exercise program together and over the next few months, Shelley started losing weight. As she lost weight, she became more popular, and she realized that the kids who had teased her now wanted to be her friends. Shelley didn't hold a grudge against them, but she is still saddened by the prejudice against overweight people.

LISA'S STORY

Lisa is a thirteen-year-old girl who began to gain weight rapidly from the age of 10 years. She had two older sisters, but Lisa was the "good kid." She never caused trouble and never complained. When she was nine, her grandmother died. Lisa was devastated, but waited till night-time to cry alone. In her room some nights, she would eat and eat in secret, and she found that eating blocked out her feelings for a while. She started gaining weight. Her parents were surprised by her weight gain, as it didn't appear that Lisa ate very much at all. They attributed the weight gain to a sluggish metabolism.

As Lisa continued to gain weight, she became more isolated from her friends, and the once fun-loving girl seemed anxious and sad. It became obvious to Lisa that eating was not solving her problems. It was only much later, when she was taken to see her pediatrician and a dietician, that she discussed her eating habits and her feelings about her grandmother. She began therapy and a healthy eating plan, and is much closer to being the happy girl that her parents and friends once knew.

Why Are Americans Gaining Weight?

The cause is not entirely simple, and as we learn more about metabolism and genetics, we realize that it is a combination of factors that lead to obesity. There is no doubt that some people are more at risk, but in general, people become overweight when they eat more calories than their bodies burn up through activity. The excess energy is stored as fat. Lifestyle behaviors related to too much intake of calories and too little physical activity are the most common causes of the recent rise in obesity. Our society has an abundance of food, which is often high in calories, beautifully presented, and tempting. In addition, we walk less, have cars at our disposal, and have to spend less energy to get our food.

The following are some of the causes of or contributing factors to obesity in young people:

- Genetics and endocrine causes
- Inactivity
- Poor nutrition
- Stress and depression
- Eating disorders (Binge-eating disorder)
- Medications

GENETICS AND ENDOCRINE CAUSES

Heredity does play an important role, with children of overweight parents having a greater risk of being overweight, although in these cases the obesity is often due to a combination of genetics and behaviors. Genetic syndromes and endocrine causes make up only a small percentage of patients with childhood obesity. These problems include Cushing syndrome and hypothyroidism, among others. Although they are rare causes of obesity, they should certainly be considered. Further studies are being done to identify the genes that may put one at risk for obesity, and hormones that play a part in determining hunger and satiety.

INACTIVITY

Many young people today are more sedentary for a number of reasons. They may spend less time doing physical activity at school. They may spend more time on the internet, playing video games, or working on the computer. Many teenagers spend excessive time watching television.

In addition, children and teens may spend less time outdoors, playing sports, or just being active in general. Unfortunately, in many schools physical education programs have been reduced or cut to make way for other programs. Parental safety concerns may also keep young children indoors more often, as neighborhoods or playgrounds may not be safe.

POOR NUTRITION

Children, teenagers and adults frequently eat "on the run." People are too busy, and there often seems to be no time to cook a healthy meal and sit down as a family for mealtimes. For children to participate in basketball, ballet and music practice while the parents juggle two jobs, something has to give. Unfortunately, what gives, too often, is quality time for the family, including the family dinnertime when everyone sits down together and catches up on events of the day. And in the long run, everyone pays a price for that.

Foods today are fast, easy, and high in sugars and fat. Quantities offered are often larger than they were in the past. In restaurants, larger portions are served. (Yes, one probably pays more.) At fast food places, super-size french-fries are offered and cups of soda are bigger. Even candy bars are larger. Many schools have fast-food outlets, and more have vending machines for candies and soda. Even some hospitals have fast-food outlets. On top of all this, on television and on billboards, one is constantly bombarded with advertisements to buy these tempting foods. Also, our social and business activities often revolve around food. Weddings, birthdays and meetings usually involve meals. Friends meet over lunch or over coffee, rather than for a walk.

STRESS AND DEPRESSION

Some people gain weight in response to certain situations or stresses, such as depression, stress at work or school, or family problems.

They may eat to fill an emotional emptiness rather than in response to hunger.

Eating Disorders

A significant percentage of people with obesity have binge-eating disorder. People with binge-eating disorder have recurrent episodes of binge eating, in which they eat very large amounts of food in a short period of time, with a feeling of being out of control over their eating. They often have failed attempts at trying to lose weight, and are often overweight. They usually have low self-esteem. Binge-eating disorder, like other eating disorders, is an illness that can have serious complications and should be taken seriously. The good news is that treatment is available. (See chapter 2 for more on binge-eating disorder.)

Medication

A less common cause of increased weight is medication. Certain medications such as steroids and some medications to treat depression and anxiety can be culprits.

Treatment

Treatment for obesity includes the following goals:

- To improve health, and avoid complications of obesity.
- To identify and treat complications if they exist.
- To increase energy.
- To increase self-esteem.
- To improve body image.
- To improve quality of life.

The first step is to make a commitment to a healthier lifestyle, which is best achieved by making gradual, long-term, healthy changes. Too many people try quick-fix diets, only to regain weight and return to their old habits soon after. You must strive for permanent, healthy changes that can last a lifetime.

After checking with your doctor, set a target weight in a healthy range. Aim to gradually decrease weight in a safe way, by eating a balanced diet and exercising regularly. Aim for health and fitness rather than only for weight loss. If you make healthy changes, you have already succeeded no matter what the scale shows.

If you are living at home with your family, involving as many family members as possible can be helpful. Together you can work on a plan to shop for healthier foods, take turns cooking healthy meals, and generally support each other.

It's important that you be ready and motivated for change. It's also important to commit to regular long-term monitoring and follow up, which will increase your chances of success.

ASSESSMENT

The first part of treatment is getting a thorough assessment by a doctor familiar with treating adolescent obesity. The assessment involves taking a detailed history, including a dietary and activity history; performing a physical examination to rule out underlying diseases or complications; and checking lab tests as indicated. If you are mildly overweight, many times you will be able to make the changes together with the help of your parents and the guidance of your primary care doctor. If you are more severely overweight, it is probably best to work with a team, which would include a nutritionist and health care providers who are very familiar with the complications of obesity, and who are able to spend the time necessary for regular monitoring and follow-up.

Treatment for the teenager who is overweight then focuses on:

- Improving nutrition
- Encouraging healthy exercise and activity
- Working on behavioral issues
- Improving self-esteem

NUTRITION

It is best to learn a healthy way of eating that can last a lifetime, rather than focusing on dieting and weight. You've heard about what happens with dieting. People restrict food for a while, and may lose weight, but then usually return to their old habits, because most diets can't be sustained. People get hungry. The main goal should be to become fitter and healthier, rather than only thinner. Children should try to achieve a healthy weight gradually. In young children this may sometimes mean a plan for maintaining their weight for a period of time as they grow in height. For older children or teenagers, or those who are significantly overweight, the aim is usually gradual weight loss in a safe manner.

A good way to become successful is by making a few specific changes at a time. You may begin, for example, by only eliminating fried foods and eating out less often. Counting calories is hard work and boring, and doesn't work well for most people. What does work is setting goals and monitoring yourself regularly.

It is important to eat a variety of healthy foods high in nutrients and fiber and relatively low in fats and sugars, and to increase intake of fruits and vegetables. Fiber, which is found in foods such as fruits, vegetables and whole grains, makes you feel full and satisfied sooner. Sadly, one teenager told me that her favorite fruits and vegetables were pizza toppings and ketchup.

Another key is to eat regularly. Skipping meals can lead to cravings and overeating later in the day. It is best to eat three meals a day with a snack or two in betwen.

Why not make one resolution today? Decide to eat a healthy breakfast every morning to give yourself energy, and to prevent hunger and cravings later in the day.

EXERCISE

Spending too much time in sedentary activities, such as watching television or playing video games, puts a person at increased risk for being overweight. An interesting study was published in the journal *Pediatrics* in May 2001 on the effects of modifying television watching and physical activity in the home. The results strongly support that television watching and the associated inactivity is related to an increased risk of obesity in children and teenagers. Parents can help by limiting television viewing to no more than one to two hours per day and discouraging eating while watching television. They can also help by promoting fitness for the whole family, and by emphasizing that exercise is important for overall health, not only for weight control. Exercise not only includes structured sports, but also unstructured activities, like taking a family walk regularly, doing yard work, or using the stairs more often. While many teenagers do participate in physical activity, many others are still too sedentary.

Are you getting enough exercise? By exercising and doing something good for your body now, you may be preventing serious health problems later.

Make the decision to limit the amount of television you watch.

Most healthy people should exercise aerobically for about thirty minutes a day at least five days a week. Any safe exercise that gets your body moving and your heart rate up is probably fine. Some teenagers enjoy participating in organized or competitive sports. This is okay as long as the sport is enjoyable and there are no excessive pressures put on you. Organized sports can teach about discipline, practice, and the importance of cooperation. On the other hand, you may prefer individual sports such as running, swimming, walking, or biking. Whatever form of exercise you do, you will feel better when you get moving.

Moderate exercise has many potential benefits, including:

- Weight maintenance or weight loss.
- Increased metabolic rate.
- General health benefits and improved fitness. (Exercise can have positive effects on heart function and blood pressure.)
- Prevention of diabetes in some people at risk.
- Improved mood.
- Stronger and more defined muscles (through strength training).
- Social benefits.
- Improved self-esteem.

People of all ages are now being encouraged to start exercising. Many symptoms and conditions that were in the past thought to be an inevitable part of growing older, are now found to be preventable with regular safe exercise. It appears that regular aerobic exercise improves health even when it doesn't cause weight loss. Also, the good news is that you don't have to do intensive exercise to see health benefits. People who walk every day have significant health benefits.

There are many ways to increase your activity level. Remember, though, that if you are starting a new exercise program it is always best to check with your doctor first. Then consider these tips:

- Ask a friend to join a gym with you.
- Make a commitment to take a walk four evenings a week with a friend or a family member.
    - Help with gardening in summer or snow shoveling in winter.
    - Take the stairs instead of the elevator.
    - Take the dog for walks.
    - Plan social events around activities such as bike rides, instead of food.

Many people wonder what is the "best" form of exercise. The answer is, any safe physical activity that you will actually do. One mom told me that she created a wonderful fitness plan for her son, in which he would be walking for half an hour five days a week. When I asked how he was doing, she said he had walked only one day that week. Why? It had rained most of the week and there was no contingency plan for rain. Also, her son did not enjoy walking. So we created a new plan in which he would play basketball outside in their yard for half an hour when the weather was good, and ride the stationary bike when it rained. He exercised 5 days the next week, and planned to get on the basketball team the next season.

Behavior Modification

Behavior modification involves identifying cues and triggers associated with eating, and teaching alternative behaviors (that is, something besides overeating) to cope with high-risk situations. It also involves changing eating patterns and learning self-monitoring. A short-term diet or exercise program is not going to work in the long run. You will regain weight if you return to your old habits. Remember, you need to find a healthier way of eating and living, one that you can enjoy, and one that can last a lifetime.

Three young teenagers told me that they had attended a weight-loss camp the prior summer. The protocol included a low-fat diet and regular exercise. The camp was far away from home, so the family was not included in this program. I asked them how it went. "Very well," they told me. They each lost between ten and fourteen pounds. "But," they added, "we put the weight back on by the fall." I don't consider that a success. A good nutrition and behavior modification plan should be one that can be continued, with adjustments if necessary. (Remember that it's always best to check with your doctor before starting any nutrition plan.)

What kinds of changes can make a positive difference in your life and health? Once you have made that commitment, here are some more changes to strive for. First you must *make a commitment to a healthier lifestyle*.

- Enlist your family for help and support.
- Aim for health and fitness rather than thinness.
- Eat a variety of foods from all the food groups to make sure that you get all the nutrients you need. You should also make sure that you drink plenty of water each day. Carrying around a plastic bottle of water can be a good reminder.
- Try to increase your intake of fiber by eating more fruits, vegetables and whole grains.
- Eat regular meals and one or two snacks every day. Try not to go longer than three to four hours without eating. Restrictive diets slow your metabolism, make you hungry and can set you up for bingeing and eating disorders. Also, they often don't work.
- Try to eat when you are hungry, rather than when you are bored.
- Eat a good breakfast every morning. This makes you less likely to develop cravings or binge later in the day.
- Have healthy food options available, and try to limit unhealthy temptations around the house.
- Eat out less often, especially at fast food restaurants.
- Try to involve your family in healthy exercise and activity.
- Limit television watching. Not only is it a sedentary activity, it constantly exposes you to snack food commercials.
- Try keeping a food journal (see below).
- Enlist the support of a close friend.

If this sounds overwhelming, start by making one or two small changes at a time. For example, you may begin by having a good breakfast every morning. Once this becomes habit, try to eat an extra fruit and vegetable every day. Later you can cut down on fats by avoiding fried foods and so forth.

Food and Activity Journals

In a food and activity journal, you record what you eat, when you eat it, and how much of it you eat.

Try to write down whether or not you were hungry before you ate each meal or snack. You also record your activity: when you exercised, what the activity was, and the duration of exercise.

Keeping a food and activity journal has several benefits. First of all, it can make you aware of how much you eat and when you eat. This is important as many people have every intention of eating healthily, but they lose track of what they have eaten. A journal can also make you aware of situations that trigger certain eating patterns.And recording activity can make you aware of how much you exercise and is often a motivator. What's more, a journal is a good form of self-discipline; it allows you (and your doctor, if necessary) to follow your progress from day to day; and it can even be fun!

When keeping a food journal, it's important to record everything as accurately as possible. Don't forget that food items such as salad dressings may add many calories, and drinks such as juices, Gatorade, cappuccinos, sodas and milk also count.

Things to Avoid When Trying to Lose Weight

This chapter has provided lots of suggestions for what to do. There are also some things you should *not* do when trying to lose weight:

Don't use very restrictive diets.

Don't use diet pills or any medications to lose weight without the advice of a physician.

Don't skip meals. This leads to hunger and cravings, and will increase the risk of bingeing.

Don't eat just because you are bored. Make a list of simple activities you enjoy doing, and do one of these the next time you are about to eat because of boredom. The urge to eat will probably pass. Examples of activities include taking a walk, drawing or painting, writing in your journal or calling a good friend.

Don't eat while watching television.

Don't be hard on yourself if you eat too much or don't eat as well as you'd like on occasion. Look at the big picture: not a short-term diet, but a lifetime of healthier eating.

Fad Diets

Unfortunately there are no magic diets that quickly let you lose weight and maintain that weight loss safely. We spend billions of dollars on diets and other gimmicks to lose weight, but most of them don't even work. Let's face it: If any of these diets worked, would there be so many of them? The only safe way to lose weight and maintain the weight loss on a long-term basis is with a sensible, healthy nutrition plan and regular exercise. I know this doesn't sound as exciting, but it works. So unless your doctor tells you otherwise, stay away from diets such as the following:

• Diets that allow only very limited types of foods, such as a "cabbage diet" or a "soup and fruit" diet.
• High protein diets that exclude or limit fruits and vegetables and carbohydrates.
• Liquid diets.
• Fasting or extremely low calorie diets.
• Diets that allow you to eat at specific times only.
• Diets specifying eating foods in certain combinations only.
• "Quick-fix" diets, such as a 7-day diet or a 2-week diet. Healthier eating should last a lifetime.

When Lifestyle Changes Are Not Enough

Medications

Sometimes weight loss medications are prescribed for people who are severely overweight. The rationale is that although these medications can have serious side effects, they may be less serious that the complications of obesity. In any case, medications should only be used under the strict supervision of a physician.

Surgery

Unfortunately, in rare cases when the above treatments fail, some patients have to resort to surgery. Surgery is rarely an option for teenagers and falls outside of the scope of this book.

In summary, although genetics and hormonal causes do play a part in obesity, the recent epidemic of obesity is almost certainly related to lifestyle. By making healthy changes in our nutrition and activity levels, we will become a healthier society. Teenagers are at a crucial stage in growth and development, and the teen years are a good time to set healthy goals for the future. The teenager who does so can set an example for the rest of society.

13

Questions and Answers

In the years that I have been taking care of teenagers, a number of questions about eating disorders and obesity have come up repeatedly. I hope the following pages will answer some of your questions too.

Q: Why is dieting a problem?

A. First of all, when I talk about dieting, I am not talking about healthy eating. I am referring to restricting foods and calories so that one is not getting adequate nutrition.

Dieting usually doesn't work. Millions of people lose weight, only to regain it right back when they go off their diet. They usually do go off the diet at some point, because most of these diets can't be sustained over a long period of time.

Not only do diets usually not work, they can also have serious medical and psychological consequences. For example:

• Young people need enough calories to grow adequately, and by restricting calories they may develop nutritional deficiencies or stunted growth.

• Lack of nutrition can lead to many other complications, including irregular or absent menstruation and osteoporosis.

• Dieting can lead to food obsessions and can increase the risk for binge eating.

• Vulnerable people who go on a diet may develop eating disorders.

• When we diet our metabolism slows down so that the body burns fewer calories. When people come off a diet, some may gain back more weight than they lost, in part because of the slower metabolism.

• Dieting and skipping meals can lead to a lack of energy.

• Dieting and poor nutrition can cause mood problems and difficulty with concentration.

• Unsuccessful dieting can lead to problems with self-esteem.

Q: Are there lab tests or studies that can definitively make the diagnosis of an eating disorder?

A: Unfortunately, there are no specific tests that point with certainty to an eating disorder. The diagnosis is made by taking a very good history and doing a good examination, and then there are a number of tests that can help in making and confirming the diagnosis. For example, abnormal electrolytes may raise suspicion that a person has been vomiting or using laxatives or diuretics.

Q: I was diagnosed with anorexia nervosa recently, and went in for a physical exam and lab tests. I was told that all my lab tests were normal. Does this mean I am okay?

A: Normal laboratory test results do not necessarily mean that everything is okay. Lab tests can be a helpful addition to a good history and physical examination, and can sometimes give us clues, or point to serious complications. However, a person can be malnourished and even have heart problems or osteoporosis and still have normal lab results.

Q: Once a patient has recovered from anorexia nervosa and weight is back to normal, are there still long-term complications to be concerned about?

A: There may be. Almost every organ system can be affected by anorexia nervosa, including the heart, the kidneys, and the immune system. In general, with early treatment, most complications can be prevented or reversed. However, especially in patients who have had anorexia nervosa for many years, we are still worried about osteoporosis (thinning of the bones). Research is still being done on brain changes in chronic anorexia.

Q: How common is osteoporosis in people with eating disorders?

A: Osteoporosis occurs more commonly in people with anorexia nervosa. Some studies indicate that it is seen in more than 60 percent of patients with anorexia nervosa and in some patients with bulimia, especially if they have a history of anorexia. It occurs in males as well as in females, and usually begins within six months of weight loss.

Q: How can osteoporosis be prevented in patients with eating disorders, and if it does occur, how is it treated?

A: The best prevention in young people is healthy nutrition, with adequate amounts of all nutrients required for optimal growth and development (including adequate intake of Calcium and Vitamin D). Through this healthy nutrition, a person should maintain a healthy weight. Another important part of prevention is moderate safe exercise, including weight-bearing exercises.

Treatment is not as easy as prevention, but it begins with following a healthy nutrition plan and regaining weight to a normal range. Safe, appropriate exercise, including weight-bearing exercise, should be part of treatment as well. Adequate intake of calcium and vitamin D is essential. Bone density tests are followed to monitor progression.

Researchers are currently studying the effectiveness of certain medications. To date, hormonal therapy has not proved effective in young people with osteoporosis related to eating disorders.

Q: Why don't we see eating disorders as often in other cultures and developing countries?

A: One of the reasons is that other cultures have not traditionally placed the same high value on appearance and thinness as we have in this culture. On the other hand we are beginning to see an increase in the incidence of eating disorders in other cultures and countries as they adopt many of the Western values. Also, because of the unfamiliarity with eating disorders in certain countries with a low incidence, when they do occur, they are not always recognized.

Q: How effective are medications such as anti-depressants in the treatment of eating disorders?

A: The treatment of a patient with an eating disorder may involve many steps or methods, medications being only one of them. The others include nutritional rehabilitation; psychotherapy: individual, group and family counseling; and education. Antidepressants may be used to treat associated problems of eating disorders, including depression. They may also be used to decrease a patient's urge to binge, and to prevent relapse among patients after weight has been restored. The antidepressant Prozac has been shown to decrease impulsive behaviors including bingeing, so it is sometimes used to treat eating disorders.

Q: *Someone told me that once you have an eating disorder, you always have an eating disorder. Is this true?*

A: This is not always the case. It is true that a certain percentage of patients will have chronic problems or recurrences, but many patients can recover fully, especially if treatment is begun early. To give one example, there are certain sports and activities that can put people at risk for eating problems. Think of the wrestlers who try to "make weight" in order to be on the team. They restrict their food intake and may develop eating problems or an eating disorder. With quick and proper intervention, they will usually recover fully.

Q: *A friend of mine was told that she has both bulimia and anorexia nervosa. Is that possible?*

A: There is a lot of overlap between the two illnesses. It is not unusual at all for individuals to switch from anorexia nervosa to bulimia, and it is less common to switch from bulimia to anorexia, so she may have suffered from both.

Q: *What is the difference between bulimia and the binge eating/purging type of anorexia nervosa?*

A: Both may have binge eating and purging, but in the second case, the person also meets the criteria for anorexia nervosa, which includes a weight of less than 85 percent of expected weight, and absence of menstruation in women who have reached menarche (the onset of menstruation).

Q: I am an 18-year-old female. I want to make sure that I am getting enough exercise, but I also want to avoid over-exercising. How can I structure a healthy exercise program?

A: It is always best to check with your doctor before beginning an exercise program. For a healthy adult, a reasonable goal would be thirty minutes of an aerobic activity five days per week, and some form of strength training on three to five days per week. (See the next question for information on weight training in children.)

Aerobic activity includes activities which increase heart rate, such as running, biking, stepping, jumping, swimming or fast walking. Always begin slowly and work up to at least thirty minutes when you can tolerate it. Listen to your body. It is normal for your muscles to feel a little tired the next day, but if you develop pain during your workout, stop, or slow down. You don't want a preventable injury keeping you from exercising for weeks or months. Thirty minutes is only a guide. Some of you, especially if you are training for an event, may exercise longer—but don't overdo it.

Strength training is best begun with light weights, gradually increased in small increments. Don't start with a weight heavier than one which you can easily lift at least ten or twelve times in a row without pain. In general, machine weights are safer, as there is less chance of lifting the weight unevenly. When starting weight training, it is essential to have proper instruction.

Q: Is weight training safe for children and teenagers?

A: Well-structured training programs can increase strength in preadolescents and adolescents. These programs, which may include the use of weight machines or free weights, can be safe in these age groups if proper training techniques and safety precautions are followed. Children and teenagers should have a medical evaluation before beginning any weight lifting or strength training program, to identify any risk factors. When beginning strength training, they should begin with no resistance or low-resistance exercises, until they have achieved proper technique. Gradually, small amounts of weight can be added. Because they are at increased risk of injury, preadolescents and adolescents should not participate in bodybuilding, power lifting or competitive weight lifting until their bones reach maturity. In general, strength training programs, which may include the use of weights, can be safe in children and teenagers if they are well-supervised and structured properly.

Q: My whole family is overweight, so I am almost resigned to the fact that I will always be overweight too. Do you think I am right to be so pessimistic?

A: It is true that genetics are very important in determining a person's risk of becoming overweight, but you still have the right to be optimistic. Even if you do have genes that may put you at risk, you will probably be able to offset that risk by modifying your lifestyle—nutrition and activity level. When families are overweight, the weight problem is often due to a combination of genetics and lifestyle factors. Have yourself evaluated by your doctor to rule out any medical causes or complications, and to help you develop a safe nutrition and exercise plan.

Q: I am currently undergoing treatment for an eating disorder. Because I was underweight, I have been restricted from doing any exercising for the past four months. When is it safe to begin exercising again?

A: It's always best to check with your doctor because each individual situation may differ. In general, though, it is usually best to restrict exercise if someone is medically unstable or significantly underweight. Sometimes exercise is reintroduced only when normal weight is approached, but at other times, moderate exercise may be appropriate if the person is stable and is gaining weight steadily. In this situation exercise can help to improve mood and increase motivation to get well. If the person loses weight, exercise should once again be restricted. Excessive exercise should never be an option for anyone.

Q: Why are eating disorders more often seen in girls?

A: It is true that girls and women seem to be at increased risk for body image concerns and eating disorders. These problems may begin to emerge as girls go into puberty. A theory is that whereas boys move more closely toward their ideal body image with more muscle mass, girls' bodies move away from what may be their ideal—that is, they may become full and curvy rather than thin. Also, our society and the media put great pressure on girls to be thin, even glorifying those who are underweight.

Although eating disorders are more common among females, the incidence among males is significant, probably at least 10 percent. Men's eating disorders may be missed, because men are less likely to present for treatment early, and even when they do, the eating disorder is not always recognized.

Q: Eating disorders run in our family. Is there anything parents can do to prevent eating disorders in their children?

A: Eating disorders may be caused by a number of factors, or the combination of them. These include genetic, neurochemical, cultural and environmental factors. Parents do have some influence over the environmental factors. It's never too early to start thinking about prevention. When children are very young, parents can already start to emphasize healthy nutrition and fitness rather than dieting and thinness. Children and teenagers should be encouraged and praised for their efforts and successes that are unrelated to appearance. An important key in the prevention of eating disorders is to help children develop a healthy body image and high self-esteem. This can be done by respecting them for who they are and making them feel valuable and loved. If parents begin to see any of the warning signs of an eating disorder, they should have their child checked as soon as possible. The earlier an eating disorder is diagnosed and properly treated, the better the outcome.

Q: I suspect a friend of mine has an eating disorder. I don't know if I would have any influence, but how can I help?

A: You can't take on the responsibility of making your friend well, but you can be supportive and caring. The other thing you can do is to encourage your friend to seek professional help as soon as possible. Your friend may deny the problem, and if you are really concerned, you may need to tell a counselor, doctor, teacher, or other trusted adult. It's not useful to be critical or judgmental. An eating disorder is a serious illness and usually needs professional treatment.

Q: How can I help my boyfriend who has an eating disorder?

A: Be supportive and caring. Let him know that you are there to help him through his treatment process, although he will ultimately be the one who takes responsibility for getting well. You can also encourage him to get professional help, since eating disorders will not usually go away on their own. Don't be critical or judgmental, and do be patient.

Q: Why do people with eating disorders so often delay seeking help?

A: Unfortunately it is true that many people with eating disorders hide their illness for weeks, months or even years before asking for help.

Some eventually ask for help themselves, and others are brought to treatment by concerned family members. In the case of bulimia and binge-eating disorder, a person may avoid going for help because of embarrassment about the bingeing and purging behaviors. In the case of anorexia nervosa, the person often denies that she is ill. She is reluctant to get well and afraid of gaining weight.

Q: If I get treated for my anorexia and begin eating more, won't I get fat?

A: With appropriate treatment and follow-up, it is very unlikely for someone with anorexia nervosa to become fat. Hopefully, you will begin to eat more regularly, reach a healthier weight range, and have less anxiety about food and weight issues. If you don't get treatment and continue to restrict your calories, it's possible you might begin binge eating; more importantly, you will be putting yourself at risk for serious complications.

Q: What is the usual outcome for patients with eating disorders, and how often do people with anorexia nervosa develop bulimia, or vice versa?

A: Although, unfortunately, some patients do have poor outcomes, for most patients who seek treatment for eating disorders, the outcome is good. About fifteen percent of people with anorexia nervosa will have developed bulimia by follow-up within a ten-year period. On the other hand, it is rare for someone with bulimia to become anorexic.

Q: Is it true that people with anorexia nervosa are never hungry?

A: Although the word "anorexia" means "loss of appetite," it is not true that patients with anorexia lack appetite. They are often hungry, but they deny their hunger and avoid food to the point of starvation because of their extreme fear of weight gain.

Q: What is the difference between someone on a strict diet and someone with anorexia nervosa?

A: A big difference between the two is that whereas a person on a diet is satisfied once goal weight is reached, the person with anorexia nervosa is never satisfied with the weight loss, and always tries to reach a lower goal weight. Also, in the case of anorexia nervosa the person is persistently preoccupied with thoughts about food, weight and shape.

Q: I have a tendency to "binge" occasionally. My weight is average, and I have never vomited. Can you recommend anything to lessen the chance of bingeing?

A: If you do have an eating disorder, and have true binge eating episodes, it is always best to get professional help. Having said that, here are a few tips to decrease the chances that you will binge.

• Eat regular meals and snacks. Having three meals a day, and trying not to go longer than four hours without eating, will lessen your chances of becoming excessively hungry and then bingeing.
• Write down a list of activities to do if you feel the urge to binge. These could include going for a walk, drawing, or taking a bath, for example.
• Exercise, in moderation, can do wonders to lift your spirits.
• Stay connected to family and friends. Don't isolate yourself.

Q: How do the media influence young girls, and is there a strong influence on boys too?

A: Frequent exposure to media images of very thin models and actresses has been shown to cause body dissatisfaction and even stress, guilt and depression among girls. Boys also seem to be sensitive to media messages. Just as body image dissatisfaction has increased among girls and young women, so too has it increased among males. The media of today show men with very muscular physiques, and advertising seems to be aimed at younger and younger people. Judging from the numbers of young men signing up for the gym and buying diet and fitness products (many of which don't work), it seems as if media images do indeed have a strong influence on males too.

Q: If the media have such a powerful effect on our culture and on the body image of young people, how can we change the media message that thinness equals beauty?

A: There are a number of things we can do to begin to change both those very powerful media messages and their influence.

- Learn to view television programs critically. Discuss with your friends or family why certain images or messages are portrayed. Could it be to sell a product, or to make people buy a fitness apparatus to lose weight?
- Be vocal and participate in discussions or presentations that promote health rather than thinness.
- Promote education about eating disorders and the harmful effects of dieting.
- Limit time spent reading fashion and fitness magazines that promote dieting and super-thin ideals.
- Emphasize qualities in people (including actors) that are unrelated to appearance. These could be personal qualities such as kindness and generosity, or they could be accomplishments.

• Consider counter-advertising—in other words, counteracting those media messages with other more positive messages.

Q: *If someone goes on a diet, does that mean they will develop an eating disorder?*

A: Not necessarily, but dieting can put a vulnerable person at risk. Some may continue dieting and lose excessive weight, and others may develop binge eating.

Q: *I have been diagnosed with anorexia nervosa, and have been trying to eat more, but I become very full and uncomfortable after eating even a small meal.*

A: Anoexia nervosa leads to starvation, and with starvation the gastrointestinal system slows down. Stomach emptying is delayed, so many people complain of fullness or bloating after eating even relatively small amounts. This symptom improves as people gradually start eating more and gaining weight.

Q: *My friend is bulimic, but her weight is in the normal range. Is she still in danger?*

A: Even normal-weight people with bulimia are at risk for some of the hidden dangers. For example: Purging, which includes vomiting or the use of laxatives or diuretics, can put one at risk for developing electrolyte abnormalities and heart rhythm disturbances. These abnormalities don't always have symptoms, and the person's weight may indeed be normal, so a bulimic person may be in danger without showing physical signs of it.

Q: What is the difference between binge eating and overeating?

A: Binge eating differs in the following ways:

- The amounts eaten are usually greater.
- There is a lack of control over the eating.
- Episodes of binge eating occur regularly.
- After the binge the person usually feels shame, guilt or disgust.

Q: Are there any serious complications associated with binge-eating disorder?

A: Binge-eating disorder can result in medical as well as psychological problems. The psychological problems include low self-esteem, anxiety or depressive symptoms, and social isolation. The medical complications are those that are seen with obesity in general, such as high blood pressure, high cholesterol, heart disease, and diabetes.

Q: Does binge eating always follow dieting?

A: No, not always. Some people begin binge eating at a young age and have no history of dieting before the first bingeing episode.

Q: What happens if someone with an eating disorder becomes pregnant?

A: Although it is not common for someone with an active eating disorder to become pregnant, pregnancy does occur. It is really ideal to get the eating disorder under control before becoming pregnant, but if a person with an active disorder does become pregnant, she should be monitored very closely throughout the pregnancy. Dieting, bingeing and purging can cause problems in both the mother and the fetus. In some cases the mother is admitted to hospital for closer monitoring and treatment.

Q: *How does one decide what form of psychotherapy would be best for someone with an eating disorder? I am sixteen years old and I have anorexia nervosa.*

A: It's always best to get specific recommendations from your own physician. In general, though, in the case of a young person with anorexia nervosa, family therapy has been found to be very effective, especially if the illness is of recent onset. Family therapy is sometimes combined with group therapy, individual therapy, or both. For an adult who is living independently, the therapy of choice might be individual or group therapy. In the case of an older adolescent or adult with bulimia nervosa, individual therapy has been shown to be beneficial. Again, this may be combined with family or group therapy in certain cases. For young patients (with any eating disorder) living with their parents, involving the family in the treatment process is very important.

Q: *Because I have an eating disorder, my parents spend a lot of time taking me to doctors' appointments and preparing meals for me. I feel very guilty, because my 12-year-old little sister often gets ignored. We never speak to her about my eating disorder, but I know that she is afraid and worries about me. I don't know what to tell her in order to make her less upset.*

A: Ask your physician or therapist for the best way to involve your sister in your treatment process. It may also be helpful to bring her to one or more of your therapy sessions. Allow her to ask questions. Brothers and sisters can help the therapist understand family interactions better, and your sister can also be a support system for you.

Q: I'm really not hungry in the morning, so I've been skipping breakfast as I'm trying to lose weight. I read everywhere that it's important to eat breakfast, but can't I save on calories if I skip it?

A: Breakfast is probably the most important meal of the day. If you don't eat something to "break the fast" of the night, your blood sugar drops, you lack energy, and you will have difficulty concentrating. Also, skipping breakfast sets you up for cravings or even binges later in the day. When too hungry, people often don't use discretion, and eat unhealthily.

Q: I am slightly overweight and am trying to eat more fruits and vegetables. There is so little time in the morning, though. Would juice do as well?

A: Juice is fine, although the whole fruit would usually be better. Fruits are more filling and provide fiber, which juice does not, and also many fruit drinks are sweetened with added sugars. Make sure you drink enough water, though.

Q: Are men also at risk for the serious complications we see in women with eating disorders?

A: Yes, men suffer similar complications. Just as in women, almost all organ systems can be affected, including the heart, kidneys, endocrine system, liver, brain and skin, among others. Men are also at risk for developing osteoporosis if they are significantly underweight.

Q: How does treatment of males with eating disorders differ from treatment of women?

A: In general, treatment is similar, but there are a few differences. The therapist needs to address the shame associated with having a disorder that was in the past considered a "female problem." Factors such as hormone changes and male body image issues also need to be addressed. It is ideal to have a health care professional familiar with some of the unique issues that concern males with eating disorders. Unfortunately, this is not always possible, as not as many males are seen in eating disorder programs, and so many physicians and therapists may still have limited experience treating them. This seems to be changing now that we are better recognizing eating disorders in males.

Q: I have an eating disorder and am not allowed to go to overnight camp this summer. I feel that I will be so much happier at camp. Does it make sense to keep me from going to camp?

A: Sometimes it does make sense. If someone has an active eating disorder and is significantly underweight or medically unstable, I think it is reasonable to forego camp. In other situations, when a person has recovered or is recovering, is gaining weight steadily, and is medically stable, it might be reasonable to go to summer camp. It would still be important to have someone there who would monitor the situation, and the camper needs to be able to return home if the eating disorder returns.

Q: I am told that I look anorexic. I am a sixteen-year-old male and although I am energetic and

feel fine, I have always been very thin. I have been
to doctors for all sorts of tests that have been
negative, and I have been told that I am well.
I wish I could put on weight, but even though
I eat very regularly, I remain thin.
Could I have anorexia nervosa?

A: It is unlikely that you have anorexia nervosa, as people with anorexia usually restrict their food intake, have an intense fear of weight gain and often view themselves as overweight in spite of being thin. It was a good idea to be checked by a physician, but try not to worry. There are some people who are genetically thin and healthy.

Q: I am recovering from an eating disorder.
Will I ever get to a point when I don't worry
about what I eat, how many calories I eat,
and when I eat? I wish I could go out to have
a meal with my friends without obsessing.

A: It does take time, but with treatment, support and patience, you will do better. As you continue to become well, you will gradually find new meaning and interest in the things around you—things that you have been oblivious to while you have been ill. As other things take on more importance, and as your values change, the obsession with weight and food will lessen.

Q: How does an eating disorder
affect relationships?

A: An eating disorder can affect all aspects of one's life, including school, work and relationships. People suffering with eating disorders often become isolated from social activities and the people around them. Their lives frequently revolve around their illness, and they become so preoccupied with thoughts about food and weight that there is little energy for anything or anyone else.

14

Conclusion

Until recently, eating disorders have been misunderstood illnesses. In addition to being thought of as disorders affecting adolescent women almost exclusively, their contributing causes and consequences were poorly understood. Fortunately, we have come to learn a lot more about these illnesses that affect not only all aspects of the sufferer's life, but also the lives of the people around them.

We have also come to learn that eating disorders affect males and females, both young and old, and know no boundaries when it comes to race, class or culture.

My hope is that awareness of eating disorders will continue to be raised in all communities. With our greater understanding of the causes of eating disorders, and with more effort aimed at prevention and early diagnosis, we will hopefully be able to prevent much of the suffering all too common among patients and their families.

Another goal should be to raise young people in such a way that they grow up with a healthy sense of self and good self-esteem.

Finally, a word to all young people: I hope that all of you will be proud of your achievements, and if you don't achieve all your goals, I hope you can be satisfied that you have tried your best. I also hope that you will take pride in who you are, be tolerant of others, and challenge the idea that appearance is in any way related to true self-worth or happiness.

Appendix A:
Quick Reference Guide

Eating Disorders

Anorexia Nervosa

Individuals severely restrict calories until they weigh less than 85 percent of their ideal body weight. They have a distorted body image and an intense fear of gaining weight and getting fat. Women who have begun to menstruate stop menstruating.

Bulimia Nervosa

Individuals develop recurrent episodes of binge eating. To compensate for the binges, they may vomit; exercise excessively; use laxatives, diuretics or diet pills; or diet between binges. Individuals with bulimia are usually of normal weight, or they may even be slightly overweight.

Binge-Eating Disorder

Individuals develop recurrent episodes of binge eating, but do not have the compensatory symptoms seen in patients with bulimia. They may have several failed attempts at trying to lose weight. They often gain weight.

Eating Disorders Not Otherwise Specified, and Other Eating Problems

Other less well-defined eating disorders and eating problems are very common and need to be taken seriously too. At this time, binge-eating disorder fits into this category, as it has not yet been formally diagnosed as a specific eating disorder.

Compulsive Exercising

Compulsive exercising may be a symptom of an eating disorder.

Body Dysmorphic Disorder

Body dysmorphic disorder is a condition that occurs in both men and women. Individuals with this disorder are preoccupied with an imagined or insignificant defect in their appearance. This causes extreme distress in some patients and can interfere with all aspects of their life. Some become severely depressed. Muscle dysmorphia or reverse anorexia may be a form of body dysmorphic disorder. This affects men almost exclusively. In spite of being large and muscular, these men imagine themselves to be small and puny, and will often work out for hours, or even resort to using anabolic steroids to try to become bigger. They are never satisfied with the degree of musculature they achieve.

A Few Basic Facts About Eating Disorders

- Eating disorders are serious, potentially life-threatening disorders.
- Eating disorders are caused by a combination of factors, including genetic, personal, family and socio-cultural factors.
- A common trigger for the development of an eating disorder is dieting. Some susceptible people who diet continue dieting and are at risk for developing anorexia nervosa. Others may go on to develop binge eating or bulimia.
- Although eating disorders occur most often in adolescent girls, they can occur in both males and females, young and old.
- Treatment is usually best done by a team of specialists with experience in the field. It involves some form of psychotherapy, nutritional counseling, and medication if needed.
- Medication is not the primary form of treatment for eating disorders, but can be useful to treat associated problems, such as anxiety or depression.

- Treatment is not easy and the road to recovery can be long.
- In spite of the above, effective treatment is available, and anyone suffering with an eating disorder should be hopeful that recovery can be achieved.

If You Think You Have an Eating Disorder

- Get professional help as soon as possible. The earlier you receive appropriate treatment, the better the outcome.
- Speak to your parents, a counselor, or your physician, to help you with a referral. You can also make use of the list of resources in Appendix B.
- Read about eating disorders so that you become more knowledgeable about their warning signs and complications, as well as the effective treatments available.
- Support groups can be helpful, but they do not take the place of treatment.
- Be hopeful. There is help available.

If Your Friend Has an Eating Disorder

- Be supportive.
- Be caring.
- Encourage your friend to get professional help.
- If necessary, tell a counselor, doctor, teacher, or other trusted adult.
- Don't be critical or judgmental.

Obesity

A Few Basic Facts

- The number of children and adolescents with obesity has risen dramatically in the last decade.
- People who are overweight have a higher incidence of medical complications such as high blood pressure, high cholesterol, heart problems, joint problems and diabetes.

- People who are overweight have a higher risk of having low self-esteem and being more socially isolated.

If You Are Overweight

- Be checked by your physician to make sure you have no complications and are safe to begin an exercise program. People who exercise regularly are more likely to keep excess weight off.
- Increase your activity level slowly, in a safe manner. Try beginning an activity such as walking or biking, and also try to introduce more activity into your daily schedule (for example, taking the stairs instead of the elevator).
- Try to eat more healthily. Start by having breakfast every morning, never skipping meals, and increasing the fiber in your diet. Dieting hardly ever works. Most people regain the weight lost and often gain more.
- Avoid eating out too often.
- Try to cut down on inactive time, such as sitting in front of the television set for hours.
- Monitor yourself, and follow up regularly as recommended by your doctor.
- Try keeping food and activity journals. They can be a good way to keep track of your eating and your exercise. They make you aware of what you do and can motivate you to change.
- Try to involve your family in healthy eating and exercise habits. It's easier if you have support.
- Remember there is no "magic" formula for weight loss.

Appendix B:
Resources

Academy for Eating Disorders
6728 Old McLean Village Drive
McLean VA 22101
(703) 556-9222
www.acadeatdis.org
   The Academy for Eating Disorders is a multidisciplinary professional orga-
nization focusing on eating disorders and related disorders.

American Academy of Child and Adolescent Psychiatry
(800) 333-7636
www.aacap.org

American Anorexia/Bulimia Association
165 West 46tl Street #1108
New York NY 10036
(212) 575-6200

American Psychiatric Association
1400 K Street NW
Washington DC 20005
(888) 357-7924
www.psych.org

American Psychological Association
750 First Street NE
Washington DC 20002-4242
(202) 336-5500
www.apa.org

Gurze Books
www.bulimia.com

National Association of Anorexia Nervosa and Associated Disorders
PO Box 7
Highland Park IL 60035
(847) 831-3438
www.anad.org

The North American Association for Study of Obesity
www.naaso.org

National Eating Disorders Association
603 Stewart Street, Suite 803
Seattle WA 98101
(206) 382-3587
www.nationaleatingdisorders.org
eating disorders information and referral help-line: (800) 931-2237

National Institute of Child Health and Human Development
31 Center Drive,
Bethesda MD 20892-2425
(301) 496-5133
www.nichd.nih.gov/

National Institutes of Health
www.nih.gov

National Mental Health Association
1021 Prince Street
Alexandria VA 22314
(800) 969-6642
www.nmha.org

Something Fishy
www.something-fishy.org

Suburban Center for Eating Disorders and Adolescent Obesity
6410 Rockledge Drive, Suite 410
Bethesda MD 20817
(301) 530-0676

Bibliography

Books

Abramson, Edward. *Emotional Eating: A Practical Guide to Taking Control.* New York: Lexington Books, 1993.

Andersen, Arnold, Leigh Cohn, and Thomas Holbrook. *Making Weight: Men's Conflicts with Food, Weight, Shape and Appearance.* Carlsbad CA: Gurze, 2000.

Basco, Monica Ramirez. *Never Good Enough: Freeing Yourself from the Chains of Perfectionism.* New York: Free Press, 1999.

Berg, Frances. *Children and Teens Afraid to Eat: Helping Youth in Today's Weight-Obsessed World.* Third Edition. Hettinger ND: Healthy Weight Network, 2001.

Boskind-White, Marlene, and William C. White, Jr. *Bulimia/Anorexia: The Binge/Purge Cycle and Self-starvation.* New York: Norton, 2000.

Bruch, Hilde. *Eating Disorders. Obesity, Anorexia Nervosa, and the Person Within.* New York: BasicBooks, 1973.

Brumberg, Joan Jacobs. *Fasting Girls: The History of Anorexia Nervosa.* New York: Vintage, 2000.

Buckroyd, Julia. *The Element Guide: Anorexia and Bulimia. Your Questions Answered.* Shaftesbury, Dorset, Great Britain. Elements Books, 1996.

Claude-Pierre, Peggy. *The Secret Language of Eating Disorders: How You Can Understand and Work to Cure Anorexia and Bulimia.* New York: Vintage, 1999.

Davis, Brangien. *What's Real, What's Ideal: Overcoming a Negative Body Image.* Center City MN: Hazelden, 1999.

Diagnostic and Statistical Manual of Mental Disorders. Fourth Edition, Text Revision. Washington DC: American Psychiatric Association, 2000.

Fairburn, Christopher, and Kelly Brownell, editors. *Eating Disorders and Obesity: A Comprehensive Handbook.* Second edition. New York: Guilford, 2002.

Gilbert, Sara Dulaney, and Mary C. Commerford. *The Unofficial Guide to Managing Eating Disorders.* Foster City CA: IDG, 2000.

Hall, Lindsey, and Monica Ostroff. *Anorexia Nervosa: A Guide to Recovery.* Carlsbad CA: Gurze, 1999.

Herrin, Marcia, and Nancy Matsumoto. *The Parent's Guide to Childhood Eating Disorders.* New York: Holt, 2002.

Hirschmann, Jane R., and Carol H. Munter. *When Women Stop Hating Their Bodies. Freeing Yourself from Food and Weight Obsession.* New York: Ballantine, 1995.

Kinoy, Barbara P., editor. *Eating Disorders: New Directions in Treatment and Recovery.* Second Edition. New York: Columbia University Press, 2001.

Kirkpatrick, Jim, and Paul Caldwell. *Eating Disorders: Everything You Need to Know.* Buffalo NY: Firefly, 2001.

Levenkron, Steven. *Anatomy of Anorexia.* New York: Norton, 2001.

Madaras, Lynda. *The What's Happening to My Body? Book for Girls.* New York: Newmarket, 2000.

Maine, Margo. *Father Hunger: Fathers, Daughters and Food.* Carlsbad CA: Gurze, 1991.

Mehler, Philip S., and Arnold Andersen. *Eating Disorders: A Guide to Medical Care and Complications.* Baltimore: Johns Hopkins University Press, 1999.

Minirth, Frank, Paul Meier, Robert Hemfelt, and Sharon Sneed. *Love Hunger: Recovery from Food Addiction—10-Stage Life Plans for Your Body, Mind and Soul.* Nashville: Thomas Nelson, 1990.

Sacker, Ira M., and Marc A. Zimmer. *Dying to Be Thin: Understanding and Defeating Anorexia Nervosa and Bulimia—A Practical, Lifesaving Guide.* Revised Edition. New York: Warner, 2001.

Sears, William, and Martha Sears. *The Family Nutrition Book.* New York: Little, Brown, 1999.

Siegel, Michele, Judith Brisman, and Margot Weinshel. *Surviving an Eating Disorder: Strategies for Family and Friends.* New York: HarperPerennial, 1997.

Wadden, Thomas, and Albert Stunkard, editors. *Handbook of Obesity Treatment.* New York: Guilford, 2002.

Zerbe, Kathryn J. *The Body Betrayed: A Deeper Understanding of Women, Eating Disorders and Treatment.* Carlsbad CA: Gurze, 1995.

Articles

Academy for Eating Disorders. "Eating Disorders and Health in Elite Women Distance Runners." *International Journal of Eating Disorders.* Wiley Publications. Nov. 2001; 30 (3).

Academy for Eating Disorders. "Parental Influences on Eating Behavior in Obese and Nonobese Preadolescents." *International Journal of Eating Disorders*. Wiley Publications. Dec. 2001; 30 (4).

American Academy of Pediatrics. Committee on Nutrition. Soft drinks replacing healthier alternatives in American diet. *AAP News*. Jan. 2002, 20 (1): 36.

Barbin JM, Williamson DA, Stewart TM, Reas DL, Thaw JM, Guarda AS. Psychological adjustment in the children of mothers with a history of eating disorders. *Eating and Weight Disorders. Studies on Anorexia, Bulimia and Obesity*. March 2002, 7(1).

Barry DT, Grilo CM, Masheb RM. Gender differences in patients with binge eating disorder. *International Journal of Eating Disorders*. January 2002, 31(1).

Byrne SM, McLean NJ. The cognitive-behavioral model of bulimia nervosa: a direct evaluation. *International Journal of Eating Disorders*. January 2002, 31(1).

Dorian L, Garfinkel PE. Culture and body image in Western society. *Eating and Weight Disorders: Studies on Anorexia, Bulimia and Obesity*. March 2002, 7 (1).

Dotti A, Fioravanti M, Balotta M, Tozzi F, Cannella C, and R Lazzari. Eating behavior of ballet dancers. *Eating and Weight Disorders: Studies on Anorexia, Bulimia and Obesity*. March 2002, 7(1).

Eisler I, Dare C, Russell GF, Szmukler G, le Grange D, Dodge E. Family and individual therapy in anorexia nervosa: A 5-year follow-up. *Arch. Gen. Psychiatry*, Nov. 1997, 54: 1025–30.

Faith MS, Berman N, et al. Effects of contingent television on physical activity and television viewing in obese children. *Pediatrics*. May 2001, 107(5).

Geist R, Heinmaa M, Stephens D, Davis R, Katzman DK. Comparison of family therapy and family group psychoeducation in adolescents with anorexia nervosa. *Can. J. Psychiatry*. March 2000, 45(2): 173–8.

Gelbaugh S, Ramos M, Soucar E, Urena R. Therapy for anorexia nervosa. *J. Am. Acad. Child Adolesc. Psychiatry*. February 2001, 40(2): 129–30.

Gual P, Perez-Gaspar M, Martinez-Gonzalez MA, Lahortiga F, de Irala-Estevez J, Cervera-Enguix S. Self-Esteem, personality, and eating disorders: Baseline assessment of a prospective population-based cohort. *International Journal of Eating Disorders*. April 2002, 31(3).

Harper, G. Eating disorders in adolescence. *Pediatrics in Review*. Feb. 1994, 15(2): 72–77.

Kaplowitz PB, Slora EJ, Wasserman RC, et al. Earlier onset of puberty in girls: relation to increased body mass index and race. *Pediatrics*. August 2001, 108(2): 347–353.

Kreipe RE, Dukarm CP. Eating disorders in adolescents and older children. *Pediatrics in Review*. Dec. 1999, 20(12): 410–420.

le Grange D. Family therapy for adolescent anorexia nervosa. *JCLP/In Session: Psychotherapy in Practice*. June 1999, 55(6).

Lemmon CR, Josephson AM. Family therapy for eating disorders. *Child and Adolescent Psychiatric Clinics of North America.* July 2001, 10(3).

Mendelson B, McLaren L, Gauvin L, Steiger H. The relationship of self-esteem and body esteem in women with and without eating disorders. *International Journal of Eating Disorders.* April 2002, 31(3).

Milos G, Spindler A, Ruggiero G, Klaghofer R, Schnyder U. Comorbidity of obsessive-compulsive disorders and duration of eating disorders. *International Journal of Eating Disorders.* April 2002, 31(3).

Pearson J, Goldklang D, Striegel-Moore RH. Prevention of eating disorders: challenges and opportunities. *International Journal of Eating Disorders.* April 2002, 31(3).

Powers PS. Eating disorders: A guide for the primary care physician. *Primary Care: Clinics in Office Practice.* March 2002, 29(1): 81–98.

Robin AL, Siegel PT, Moye AW, Gilroy M, Dennis AB, Sikand A. A controlled comparison of family versus individual therapy for adolescents with anorexia nervosa. *J. Am. Acad. Child Adolesc. Psychiatry.* Dec. 1999, 38(12): 1482–9.

Stettler N, Zemel BS, Kumanyika S, Stallings VA. Infant weight gain and childhood overweight status in a multicenter, cohort study. *Pediatrics.* Feb. 2002, 109(2).

Vandereyckenn W, Van Vreckem E. Brothers and sisters: How they can help you recover. *Eating Disorders Today.* Spring 2002 1(1).

Zipfel S, Reas D, Thornton C, Olmsted MP, Williamson DA, Gerlinghoff M, Herzog W, Beumont PJ. Day hospitalization programs for eating disorders: A systematic review of the literature. *International Journal of Eating Disorders.* March 2002, 31(2).

Index